MuscleBuilding For EveryBody

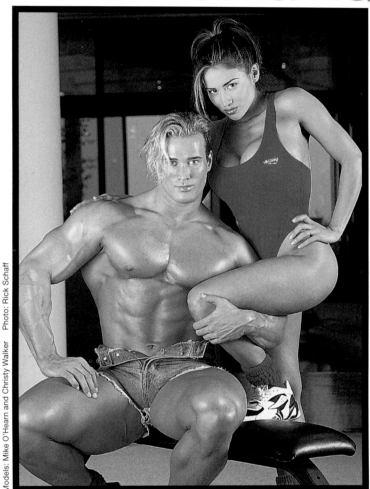

Models: Mike O'Hearn and Christy Walker   Photo: Rick Schaff

Training & Nutrition to Develop a Muscular Body
By Robert Kennedy

Copyright 2002 By Robert Kennedy

Published by MuscleMag International
5775 McLaughlin Road
Mississauga, ON
Canada L5R 3P7
www.emusclemag.com

Designed by Jackie Thibeault
Edited by Sandy Wheeler

Canadian Cataloguing in Publication Data

Kennedy, Robert, 1938-
    Musclebuilding for everybody : training & nutrition to develop a
muscular body/by Robert Kennedy.

ISBN 1-55210-025-1

    1. Bodybuilding. 2. Bodybuilders--Nutrition. I.Title.
II. Title: Muscle building for everybody.

GV546.5.K456 2002   646.7'5   C2002-902134-0

Distributed in Canada by
CANBOOK Distribution Services
1220 Nicholson Road
Newmarket, ON
L3Y 7V1

Distributed in the United States by
BookWorld Services
1933 Whitfield Park Loop
Sarasota, FL 34243

Printed in Canada

Introduction

How do you like the body you were born with? Not too bad, but you would definitely like to improve it? Most people feel the same way. Well, if you are over 20 you can forget about increasing your height, your hairline or your facial features. But there is good news. You can drastically change your appearance in a positive manner – by building up your muscles. Muscularity is the one factor you can influence in a positive way for tremendous changes. The addition of muscle brings with it a double benefit: Musclebuilding not only dramatically improves your appearance, it also gives your health a tremendous boost. In fact there is almost nothing as beneficial for your body as building up the muscles.

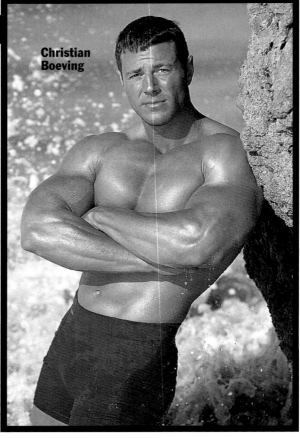

Christian Boeving

When we speak of building up the muscles, we are referring to the entire process – from mental preparation to nutrition and training to postworkout recovery. Musclebuilding is a positive process and you will enjoy the results it provides. Whether you are male or female, new to the world of musclebuilding or a seasoned bodybuilder looking to move to the next level, *MuscleBuilding for EveryBody* will provide the insight you need to make positive change to your physique.

Musclebuilding Benefits

Covert Bailey, the famous fitness guru, relates the benefits of "King Muscle," which include the improvement of blood cholesterol, lowering blood pressure, burning fat, hardening bones, thinning blood, reducing stress, and speeding up the metabolism. And these are just a few of the more notable health benefits that building up the muscles provides. The appearance of the body is radically enhanced by musclebuilding. It is easy to see why – the male physique is roughly half muscle, the female slightly less. By altering this large portion of the body you can literally change your shape. Softness becomes hard. Straight becomes curved. As Tormont Webster's *Illustrated Encyclopedic Dictionary* points out, "The shape of the body is defined largely by the striated muscles, which form by far the greatest part of the body's muscle tissue." The shape of the skeletal muscles (or lack thereof) sets the standard for the appearance of the human body. You can use this factor to your benefit in improving your appearance.

The male physique is roughly half muscle, the female slightly less.

One of the most fascinating aspects of muscle is that it readily responds to stimuli. The human body is not static – it is in a constant state of change. That's right – your body is always changing. And one of the most active areas is the muscle system. Muscle responds strongly to challenge. Repeated stimulation brings about obvious visible changes in musculature. These changes can come fairly quickly, particularly if the stimulation is significant. Human muscle will respond by adapting and becoming bigger, tougher, and stronger to handle that challenge – and then some.

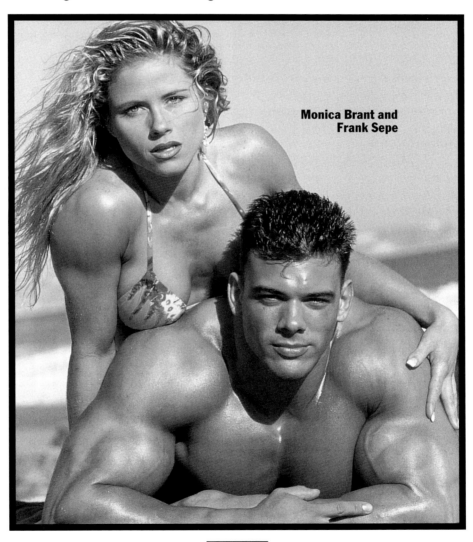

Monica Brant and
Frank Sepe

Muscles involve action. Consider a classic dictionary definition of *muscular* – "pertaining to or consisting of muscle or muscles. Accomplished with or involving the use of muscles; having strong muscles." Using an analogy

Muscles respond to challenge by adapting and becoming bigger, tougher and stronger.

from the plant world, muscles bloom when they are worked; they wilt when they are not used. Most people know what happens when someone has an arm or leg in a cast for a few weeks. The limb atrophies down to a spindly shape, while the free limb remains stout and strong. Inactivity is the bane of muscle tissue; activity is what keeps it going. Although gravity does provide some toning effect, that alone is not enough to keep the human muscle system functioning – activity is also required. Ask anyone who has worn a cast for any length of time.

Musclebuilding is no longer a case of simply exercising and watching the muscles grow. This elementary approach will produce some limited results. However, the training of muscles has quickly become a complex endeavour. Scientific means have been brought to bear on the human muscle system, and the resultant studies have provided a variety of systems available to utilize for the best results. The past five decades have been revolutionary in our understanding of training the muscles. And in addition to research on training systems, much insight has been gathered on nutrition and the role various nutrients play in enhancing the muscles (or detracting from them if not provided).

This book is intended to help you increase your muscularity. This translates into a direct increase in both muscle size and strength. Whether you need to build a more powerful body to become better conditioned for sports, or simply want to look and feel better, *MuscleBuilding for EveryBody* will provide you with the tools you need to wage a successful war against laziness, sedentary living, aging and complacency – the

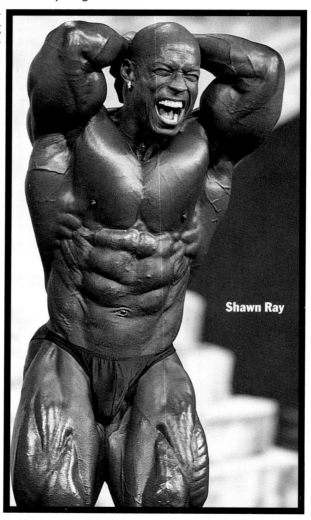

Shawn Ray

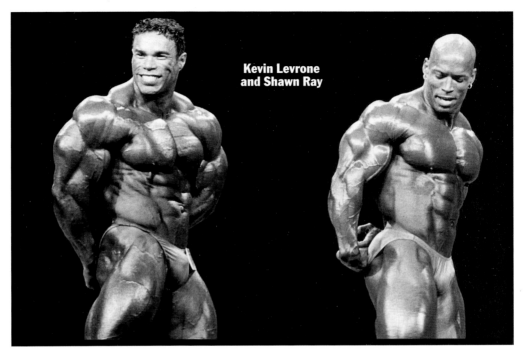

Kevin Levrone
and Shawn Ray

Never use excuses like "I can't" or "It's too hard" – Shawn Ray

forces that sink most of the population into fat and unhealthy mediocrity. The answer to modern society's physical ills (and many of their mental ones as well) is muscle.

MuscleBuilding for EveryBody also provides the tools you will need to take your body to the next level. I will start with the basics and then step up to the most modern and advanced approaches for getting more out of your muscles. The sources for this insight include the best musclebuilding champions on the planet, as well as scientific and sports researchers who focus on empirical results to define what works and what doesn't.

If you want to change your body fast, zoom in on your muscles. There is no better vehicle for rapid body change than to challenge the muscles. And when you do, bring your best to the gym. Make no mistake – the muscles don't change their shape without some effort. Shawn Ray, one of the elite physique stars of the modern era, points out that you should never use excuses like "I can't," "It's too hard," "It's too heavy," "It's my light day" or "Take it easy." Ray approaches his training with hardcore desire and strong inner motivation – totally ablaze with fire and desire to be the best. That type of attitude is exactly what is required to make the muscles conform to your desire for change. So bring into action the best tools for the job of making your muscles the best they can be. Enjoy the challenge.

BUILDING A FIRM
FOUNDATION

The most crucial element of any structure is its foundation. It is not wise to build a house on sand. Likewise, it is not wise to use a flimsy component such as cardboard to support an entire building. The foundation must be firm enough to hold everything else to be built upon it. This concept is also true for increas-

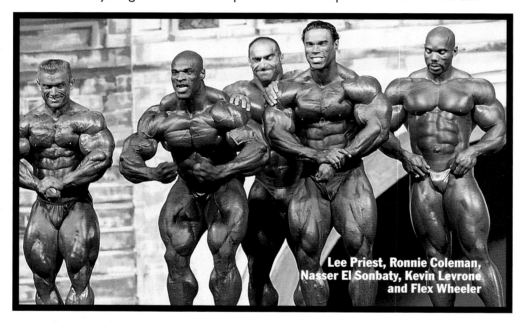

Lee Priest, Ronnie Coleman, Nasser El Sonbaty, Kevin Levrone and Flex Wheeler

ing the musculature of the human body. You must first build a firm foundation. Work to establish key basic-training principles before going on to advanced movements and techniques that are meant for shaping the body. Advanced techniques work great – but only if there is a basic foundation already established.

Building a solid physical foundation will give you the necessary base for all further physical developments. Some people make the mistake of trying to emulate the advanced finishing movements used by the professionals before they have any real foundation to build on. The outcome of this mistake is, they don't see the results they expect and are often prone to quitting at this point, believing that resistance training doesn't really work for them. The problem lies not in the resistance training but in the approach chosen. So avoid this common mistake and put off the more advanced techniques until you have mastered the basics. Of course if you currently have a good base, you can move on to the chapters featuring the advanced training techniques.

You may or may not have actually built a good foundation. In either case, it is always wise to return to the basics frequently to ensure the soundness of your training and to recharge the muscle bellies of each major muscle group.

Muscle training guru Dr. Ollie McClay makes a focus on the basics as an essential part of training anyone he works with and he mixes basic movements into virtually all sessions. Why? Because the basics bring about the most results in the shortest amount of time. Once you have the basics, the advanced techniques will prove fruitful.

Yes, build a strong foundation. That's the best way to start your body down the path to a new physique. And it may come quickly. Lee Priest, a tremendously built Australian, gained very significant muscle size after only eight months of weight training.

Recruitment Patterns

A crucial aspect of building a proper foundation requires the involvement of the central nervous system in training. Bruce Craig, PhD, from the Human Performance Laboratory at Ball State University, notes in *Strength and Conditioning Journal*, "Exposing the central nervous system (CNS) to a new experience sets up a recruitment pattern that produces enough force to move the muscle." Translated, more than just your muscles are involved in moving the weights around when you train. Your nerves also play a central role and it is a good idea to spend time building a basic foundation that pulls both the neural networks and the connected muscles.

Research even indicates that the first gains in training are neurological. The muscle gains will follow, provided the stimulation is constant. That's why people who have trained before make such rapid returns to previous levels compared to those who have never trained — the neural networks and muscles have all been down that road before, and soon get back to where they had been. Time spent on the basics is never wasted and is essential before moving on to the next level of musclebuilding.

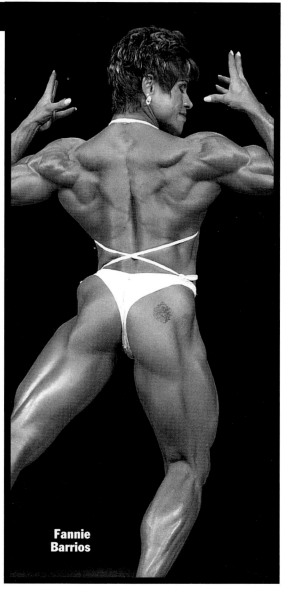

Fannie Barrios

Learning the Overload Principle

Central to building the muscles up is the overload principle. The human skeletal muscles grow to a certain level and then taper off due to the fact that daily living does not challenge them very much. To move beyond the average level, the muscles need to face an "overload." The use of overload principles is common among training athletes, as noted by the National Strength and Conditioning Association's Basic Guidelines:

"During the past two decades, the effectiveness of carefully planned weight-training programs as a method of improving body development and sports performance has been accepted on the basis of scientific literature. Significant benefits can be gained from the systematic and proper application of resistance-training principles, which are based on scientific investigation. The overload principle remains one of the primary tenets of resistance training; according to the principle, the demands on the neuromuscular system are progressively increased over the training period ... Resistance training provides

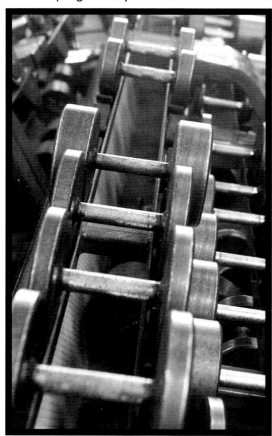

When building a basic foundation, the choice of exercise is very important.

one of the most potent and effective exercise stimuli available for athletes to increase muscular performance capabilities. In addition, the associated adaptations to resistance training contribute to improved sports performance and prevention of injury."

This increase in the demands on the muscles via the weights is the ultimate manner in which to make the muscles grow. How are the demands on the muscles increased beyond those associated with daily living? Weights are used to allow a balanced and incrementally more demanding stimulus. Translation, the weight bar, dumbells and machine allow for an orderly increase in workload to be applied to the movement, allowing the muscles to gradually adapt to the challenge — and in turn get bigger. In this process of gradually manipulating the muscles to become larger and stronger, five acute training variables are brought into play — choice of exercise, order of exercise, volume, load and rest. Each aspect plays a very important part in the production of "bigger and badder" muscles.

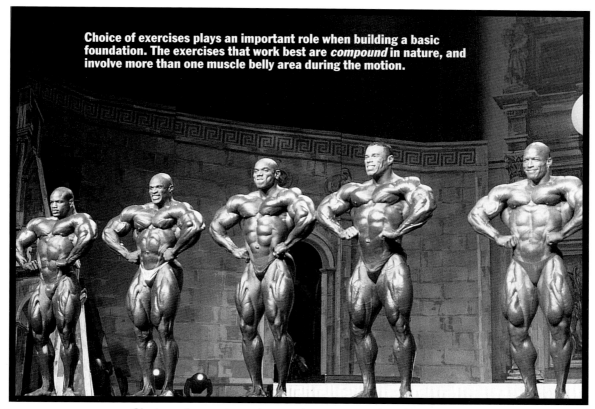

Choice of exercises plays an important role when building a basic foundation. The exercises that work best are *compound* in nature, and involve more than one muscle belly area during the motion.

Choice of exercises plays an important role when building the foundation. The exercises that work best are *compound* in nature, and involve more than one muscle belly area during the motion. The basic exercises hit the larger muscle groups of the body in a fairly simple scheme that triggers muscle growth as well as the metabolism. A select few basic exercises are head and shoulders above the rest for producing initial results – the squat, an overhead pressing movement, the bench press, the bent-over row, the triceps pushdown and an exercise incorporating the curl movement. Include these exercises in any basic training program to make it a success. They hit the muscles straight on – and make them grow.

The Squat

The squat is the essential body-shaping tool. It acts as a metabolic optimizer, placing great demand upon the body's largest muscle group, the quadriceps. The squat lets you find out right away that building the muscles up is not a task for the faint-hearted. Notice the grimace on the face of anyone who is squatting! The squat is so tough because it demands total involvement – mind and muscles working together. And in return it rewards you – it is one of the top exercises for creating postworkout fat-burning, kicking the metabolism into high gear, and

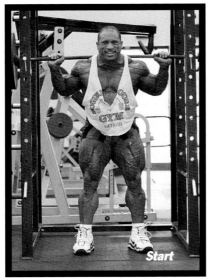

Start

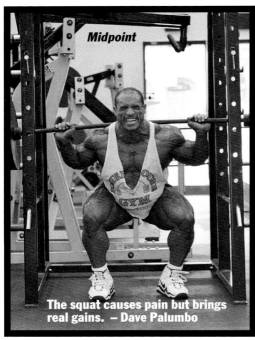

Midpoint

The squat causes pain but brings real gains. — Dave Palumbo

influencing the growth of muscles throughout the body – including the main target, the thighs. The squat is also nasty because it is the supreme free-weight motion and the ultimate lifting tool. Consider the insight of Nasser El Sonbaty on the use of hardcore free weights:

"Everyone who is honest will admit he prefers machines over free weights because machines are more convenient and cause less muscle pain. They require less concentration and are generally less dangerous. But if you want real gains you must train hard and heavy. You must always choose the least favorite exercises to actually get the best possible results. So go for the least favorite exercises, the free weights ... and go for the muscle pain!" The squat causes pain – no way around that. It causes pain but brings real gains.

The squat is done by placing a barbell across the back and squatting down (hence the name) to a position where the thighs are roughly parallel with the floor. Then push the weight back up. You must keep the shoulders level and the body balanced throughout the movement. Elevating the heels slightly (1 to 2 inches) will help put the emphasis of the movement on the thigh muscles, as will taking a narrower stance. Your eyes should be focused upward during the exercise to help you stay balanced. The load should be heavy enough that the final few repetitions are very difficult to complete. However, if you are totally new to the squat. In that event you should use a light weight for the first couple of workouts to learn the motion and let your body become accustomed to the neuromuscular recruitment patterns involved in the squat. A *repetition* is one full movement from beginning to midpoint, back to beginning. A *set* is a group of several repetitions performed in one nonstop segment. For the squat, one rep involves moving from a standing position to the parallel position, then back up again.

Without any noticeable rest, the movement is repeated. Do 2 sets of 8 to 10 repetitions during the first month of training; thereafter increase to 3 sets of 8 to 10 reps.

The Overhead Press

The press motion is a close competitor with the squat for the ultimate muscle-challenging movement. The reason is, if the full movement from the floor is used, more muscles are recruited than with any other exercise. There are several variations of the overhead press – seated, standing, behind the head, dumbell, and Olympic-style movements such as the push-press. Start with the standard overhead press, also known as the military press. Using a grip slightly wider than shoulder width, pick a barbell up off the floor and lift it to shoulder level (this motion is called a "clean"). The barbell should come to rest by your upper chest region. From this point the motion is then a simple upward push. Press the bar up until your arms are fully extended overhead, hold for half a second, then lower to the chest/neck area. Repeat for 2 sets of 8 to 10 repetitions, adding a third set about three to four weeks into your training.

The "clean" involves more muscles than any other exercise.

The overhead press involves several muscle groups but the main recipient of the action is the shoulders, known as the deltoids. Shawn Ray, owner of a super pair of shoulders, states, "Big, round deltoids definitely set off the symmetry of your entire physique." He is correct – well-developed shoulders definitely add to the shape of the body.

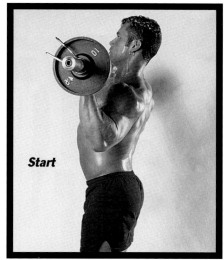

Start

The overhead press involves several muscle groups but the main recipient of the action is the shoulders.

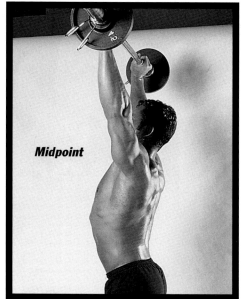

Midpoint

The Bench Press

The bench press is unique in that it is done from a prone position. A barbell is placed on the rack attached to a bench. From the prone position, the barbell is lifted off the rack and lowered until it touches the chest area. Once the bar touches the chest it is pressed back up to a full extension of the arms. As with the overhead press, the hand placement should be slightly wider than shoulder width. The downward stroke of the bench press motion should be slow to moderate in speed to allow for a light touch down. Do not bounce the bar off your chest. The bench press will really blast the muscles of the upper body. Do 2 sets of 10 to 12 reps initially, then advance to 3 sets of 8 to 10 after your first month of training.

The Bent-Over Row

The thighs are the biggest muscle group in the entire body. Guess which group is the biggest in the upper body? If you guessed the back, you are correct. The back muscles make up the largest area of the upper body and it takes a tough exercise to challenge them. The bent-over row is just such an exercise. This movement is done by bending forward at the waist and grasping a barbell with a medium-width grip. The barbell is then rowed upward until the it

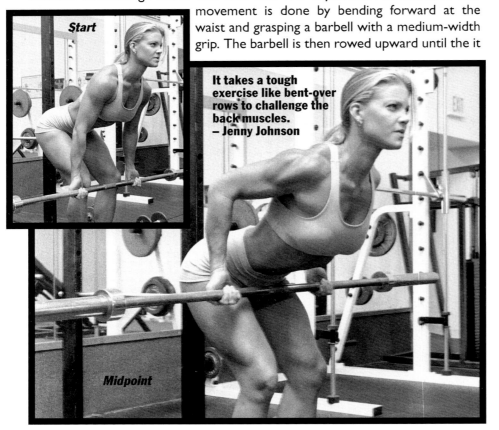

Start

It takes a tough exercise like bent-over rows to challenge the back muscles.
– Jenny Johnson

Midpoint

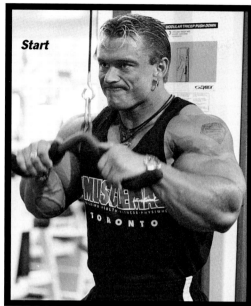

Start

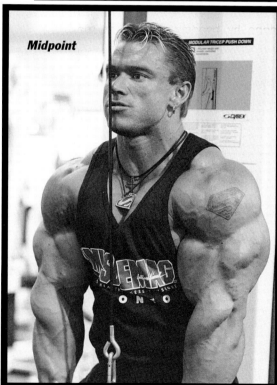

Midpoint

**The triceps cable pushdown is
a superb triceps training tool.
– Lee Priest**

touches the body at about the level of the upper ribs. The elbows should move out and back at the top of the lift. Touch the bar lightly to the body, then lower it all the way down and repeat. Use moderate speed. Bend forward to do the exercise, but do not lock the knees; keep them slightly bent to take some of the pressure off the lower spine area. The bent row motion works on both depth and breadth of the upper back. Do a couple of sets of 8 to 12 reps per workout for a month, then move on to 3 sets.

The Triceps Pushdown

The triceps pushdown is a movement done on a cable-pulley apparatus, which isolates the action to just the triceps. Grasp the pulley handle (bar or rope) and press downward (which will in turn push the attached weight plates upward). The key to good stimulation here is to use solid form. Keep the elbows in as close to the sides of the body as possible, and don't lean forward. Do not use your bodyweight to push the bar downward; make the triceps do all the work. The triceps cable pushdown is a superb training tool. As multi-Mr. Olympia Dorian Yates points out in his book *Blood and Guts*, "I've tried every triceps exercise imaginable and the best two I've found for packing on serious beef are cable pressdowns and lying EZ-curl extensions."

When doing the triceps pushdown, do not try to push down massive amounts of weight initially; instead focus on the form of the movement and *feeling* the muscles work. Another tip – don't rest at the top or bottom. Keep tension on the triceps. Constant tension throughout the movement is a key to stimulating new muscle growth.

The Curl

The barbell curl is a power movement that calls into play the biceps muscles of the upper arm. This lift is done by grasping a barbell with roughly a shoulder-width hand placement, palms facing upward. Curl the weight up to the neck area in an arc motion while keeping the elbows stationary by the sides of the body. Keep the elbows there – that is vital. Most beginners make the mistake of letting the elbows drift forward as the movement is done, taking the stress off the biceps, and negating the exercise. The elbows should always be pointed down, not out. Additionally, lower the bar back to the starting point with a slow to moderate speed. Avoid the novice tendency to bounce the bar off the thighs.

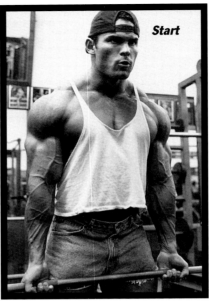

Start

Curls can be done with a barbell or dumbells, or on a cable pulley machine. There are many types of curling exercises and related motions such as the preacher curl and Zottman curl. In the initial stages of training you should focus on the basic barbell curl, which hits the biceps hard. The barbell curl is a staple for arm size and power. Do 2 sets of 8 to 10 repetitions for a month, then increase the range to 3 sets. Use a weight that makes your biceps really burn for the final 2 or 3 reps, but maintain good form to the end.

Strong & Simple

That's it for the first workout program. One of the biggest mistakes people make in entering the musclebuilding arena is trying to do too much too soon. The result is an early exit from the program. Indeed, most gym owners note that the vast majority of new members don't last beyond three months. Instead of trying to do every exercise imaginable, one should focus

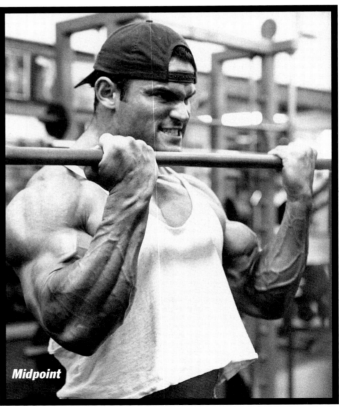

Midpoint

Avoid the tendency to bounce the bar off the thighs when performing barbell curls. – Matt Duvall on the basics – the squat, overhead press, bench press, bent-over row, triceps pushdown and barbell curl. This routine involves virtually all of the major muscle groups and these movements can be easily learned.

Initial Workout Schedule

Squats	2 sets	8-10 repetitions
Overhead presses	2 sets	8-10 repetitions
Bench presses	2 sets	10-12 repetitions
Bent-over rows	2 sets	8-10 repetitions
Triceps pushdowns	2 sets	10-12 repetitions
Barbell curls	2 sets	8-10 repetitions

Use this routine twice a week for the first month of training. Stretch and go through the motions of the movements before you actually do them. If you happen to be over the age of 40, run the idea of resistance training past your physician to get the green light in the event you happen to currently have complications that may require moderation in applying the workout. Otherwise, get to work!

Second Phase

Squats	3 sets	8-10 repetitions
Overhead presses	3 sets	8-10 repetitions
Bench presses	3 sets	10-12 repetitions
Bent-over rows	3 sets	8-12 repetitions
Triceps pushdowns	3 sets	10-12 repetitions
Barbell curls	3 sets	8-10 repetitions

After the first month, increase to 3 sets per exercise. This will intensify the workload on the muscles to stimulate new growth.

Repetition Range

The number of repetitions per set should be in the range of 8 to 12. There is a reason for this. If too many repetitions are done, the direction of the workout changes from musclebuilding to endurance. Endurance is a fine endeavor, but it is not the aim here, neither is attempting to make a one-rep maximum lift. This specific range of 8 to 12 reps has been found (via empirical means) to best support the goal of building up the muscles. Look at the routines used by the top bodybuilders – Ronnie Coleman, Lee Priest, Dexter Jackson, Jay Cutler, Juliette Bergman, Vickie Gates, etc. – the reps fall into a consistent range. And the same holds true for the top bodybuilders of the past decades as well. Arnold, Lee Haney, Dorian Yates, all used a similar rep range. Certainly they deviate from the usual at times, but in general they go with the specific range of 8 to 12 reps per set for building the muscles up.

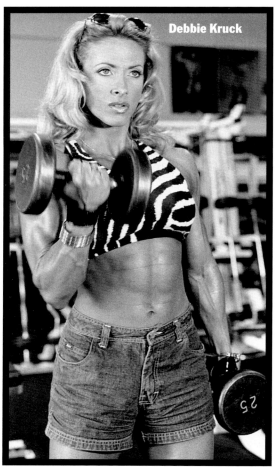

Debbie Kruck

Scientific studies have found that, for working the muscles for specific responses, the repetition ranges fall into three basic areas. Most research has revealed that poundages which allow for 6 or fewer reps (as a comparison to one-rep maximum capability) provide the most strength and power benefits. Weight loads based on 6 to 12-repetition maximums provide moderate power, strength and endurance gains but the best muscle size (hypertrophy) gains. Finally, weight loads that allow 20 or more repetitions to be performed nonstop primarily enhance muscular endurance capability with no real strength gain. (The one exception is the 20-rep squat, which has been shown to increase both size and strength.)

Peter Nielsen, a personal trainer, natural bodybuilder, and holder of more than 70 titles, splits out the repetition range in roughly the following manner in his book *Will of Iron*:

"Here are the basic principle of reps … Is strength all you want? Do you want to bulk up? Then pure unadulterated anaerobic exercise is the ticket. Look at 8 repetitions as a long set … Is definition and endurance your goal? You want to get your musculature cut or ripped? Then you're looking at basic sets of about 15 reps. For me, 10 is a magic number. A set of 10 reps builds strength and muscle, but it also builds up definition. In any basic program, think of sets as 10 reps each. Muscles that need more work get more sets. Ten reps is a number infinitely more important than the number of pounds you are moving. Gauge it this way. No matter what movement you are making – the eighth, ninth and tenth reps *should be* difficult (to the point where an eleventh might not be possible, or only with utmost effort). When you fit that formula, the amount of work you are doing is right for that muscle."

Nielsen likes exactly 10 repetitions, others like 8 or 12 reps to stimulate muscle hypertrophy. If you are in this general range you will make the best progress, provided the amount of weight you use strongly challenges the muscles for the final 2 or 3 repetitions. Incorporate a range of 8 to 12 repetitions for each set, so you can build the muscles up in the most rapid manner.

Commit this formula to memory:

Muscle power & strength = 1-6 repetitions
Muscle size (with power & strength) = 6-12 repetitions
Muscle endurance = 20+ repetitions

As mentioned, the best range is 8 to 12 repetitions, as this allows for increases in both strength and muscle size. Once you have a year or so of training under your belt it will be fine to mix in occasional sets with a lower repetition range for a focus on strength, or to increase the rep range once in a while. However, for beginners and as a good baseline, stick with the recommended 8 to 12 repetitions.

Number of Sets

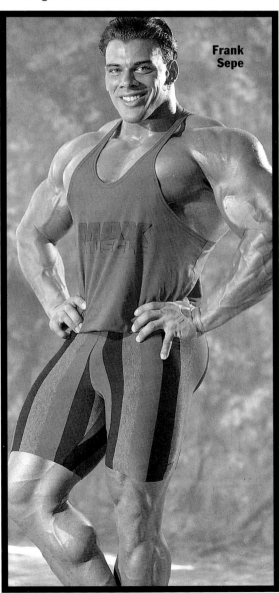

Frank
Sepe

How many sets should you do? Initially follow the recommended 2 sets per exercise for the first month of training and 3 sets thereafter. As your body becomes accustomed to the training program, you will move up from a single exercise per bodypart to two or three exercises per bodypart. Each exercise will be performed for 1 to 3 sets. Several sets can be done for major muscle groups.

There is always the chance that your physique will be the exception to the rule and a different set or repetition range will actually spark better muscle gains for you. If so, then go with the flow. One of the keys to building solid and sizeable muscle is to go with what works. You will need to experiment. However, give the basic training program some time (approximately 8 to 12 months) to get your body conditioned, to establish the neuromuscular pathways, and to acquire the basic coordination necessary for long-term success before you branch out into the more advanced realms of bodybuilding. Learn to crawl before you walk and put in some time building a foundation that is solid and strong.

"No-Mo"

One of the most deadly enemies of anyone who trains is momentum. In most sports momentum is a plus. However, in building the muscles momentum is a negative factor. Why? At any given time in a weightlifting motion one of two forces is moving the weight – momentum or muscle. If momentum is moving the weight, the muscles are not being worked to maximum. In fact they are

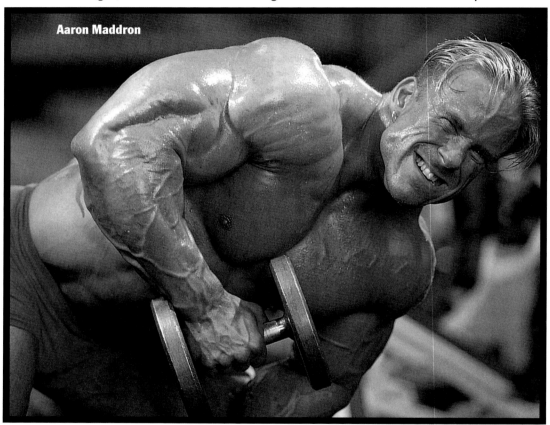

Aaron Maddron

being robbed of their training time. Momentum is built up by the speed of the movement of the weight and by body placement. Bouncing the bar, heaving it up, swinging back the elbow joint – are all typical momentum plays. Olympic lifters use momentum on purpose – but their aim is not to build muscle, but to heave up as much weight as possible. For musclebuilding momentum is undesirable.

Using momentum is often referred to as *cheating*. If someone is said to have cheated the weight up, it's because they have used momentum to help make the lift. This often occurs when a weightlifter is trying to set a new record. Unfortunately cheating often leads to injury. Three other forms of cheating are arching the back when bench pressing, swinging the dumbells up for laterals, and failing to complete the full range of motion in any exercise movement. Result?

The muscles are cheated. They don't get the stimulation they need in order to grow.

The opposite of cheating is the use of good form. From Arnold Schwarzenegger to Dorian Yates to Paul Dillett, all the top physique stars credit discipline – the consistent use of good form when lifting weights. Dorian Yates even goes so far as to call good form the key to bodybuilding success. As he notes in *Blood and Guts,* "People who use bad form are concerned with how much weight is on the bar. Instead they should be concerned with how much stress is being put on the muscle to make it work hard and grow … I suggest increasing your poundage only if you can put more stress on the muscle you want to work."

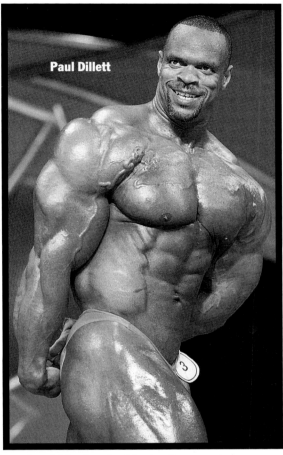

Paul Dillett

One of the most important factors in good form is *proper body alignment.* For standing movements such as the squat, barbell curl and press make certain to have the spine and shoulders in place. The shoulders should be level with the floor and the spine should not be bent unnaturally. Also avoid tilting to either side as this is an open invitation for injury. Leaning to one side when squatting can cause a major back injury. Always focus on keeping the spine centered and square. When doing seated and prone movements avoid arching your back to avoid injury to the spine.

Always start a new exercise with a relatively light weight. Allow your body to become familiar with the movement. The muscles and nerves need to get acquainted with the motion before you load up the weight and put on the heavy-duty pressure. By learning the basic range of motion of a movement with a light weight, you prepare the body for when you do crank it up and go heavy. Never start a new exercise by trying to max out. Save the heavy stuff for later. And remember, heavy weights don't always build muscle, especially if they are not used correctly. A lighter weight applied directly to the muscle is much better than a heavier weight that is misapplied.

Make sure to warm up before getting into the meat of the workout. A few minutes to bring the body up to speed before hitting the intense stuff is time well spent. And go through the motions of each movement without the weights to help get you going.

Training Safety

In addition to using proper form, take further safety precautions. Heavy metal has no mercy. Drop a plate on your toe and you'll discover a whole new level of pain. If possible, use a spotter when doing prone movements such as the bench press, and for heavy lifts such as the squat. A spotter is a person who watches your lift and is ready to assist if you get in trouble. For very heavy squats and bench-press movements, sometimes you need two spotters. If you work out alone in a gym and are planning a heavy lift, it is a good idea to ask another gym member to spot you. And always be willing to return the favor. Weights are dangerous and the more risk you can eliminate from the workout the better. However, don't be a baby and let little bumps and bruises

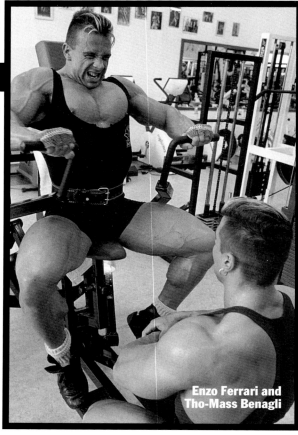

Enzo Ferrari and Tho-Mass Benagli

deter you. The gym is no place for pussycats – you need a tough mental and physical approach that keeps on coming through thick and thin.

Wear loose sweats that allow ease of full body movement. Wear a pair of shoes with good tread that allows your feet to get a firm grip on the floor. The last thing you want to have happen is to slip while you're carrying a heavy load in your arms or on your back.

Warning: there are three times when weightlifting is more dangerous than normal – when you are new to the gym, when you have been training to a degree where you have become cocky, and when you are trying a heavy one-repetition maximum lift. Be aware of these three *danger zones* – beat the odds and pay particular attention to your training form at these times to avoid injury. Although weight training can be dangerous, you can avoid injury by using strict form and good common sense.

Choosing a Gym

Where should you work out to build your muscles? Most people have two basic choices – the local gym or a home gym. Both have pros and cons.

Gym cost per month	Initial fee	Overall cost for 10 years	Overall cost for 20 years	Overall cost for 30 years
$25	$100	$3,100	$6,100	$9,100
$40	$100	$4,900	$9,700	$14,500
$60	$100	$7,300	$14,500	$21,700
$75	$100	$9,100	$18,100	$27,100
$100	$100	$12,100	$24,100	$36,100

Monthly payments to the local gym of anywhere from $25 to $100 or so may not seem like much but they add up. Over the course of several years the cost can be substantial. Purchasing equipment and working out at home is more expensive in the short-term but much cheaper in the long run. You can buy a nice Olympic set, benches, a couple of machines, and dumbells for a lot less than it costs for continuous gym use over an extended period of time. However, there are other considerations. Some people like the sense of community at the local gym, and the great variety of machines available. Those who work out at home may like the quiet atmosphere and the freedom to train whenever they want to.

There are good reasons to choose either side, depending on individual personal needs. If you do choose to go with a home gym, the second bay in a garage often works well. The floor is solid and the ceiling high. Some people like to put down a 1/2-inch rubber mat to cushion the weight against the floor. Don't get chintzy. Put out a few dollars and get the better equipment. Go for 2- or 3-inch tubing on the bracing. A couple of very useful pieces of equipment are the leg sled/press, squat rack, cable pulldown/rowing apparatus, and you'll need a solid bench press stand.

If you decide to join a gym, choose one that has heavy-duty weights and an ample number of machines. Make sure it is open both early and late. Forget the chrome plates and mirrors – they are usually tilted toward the aerobics crowd. And don't necessarily sign up at the *closest* gym. That may not be the best deal – it's worth driving a bit further if you get in a good workout.

Training Partner?

Should you train with a partner or go solo? If you are planning to lift heavy weights a spotter is a real plus. A partner can also provide added insight to your training, keep an eye on your form (or lack of it), and make suggestions for improvement. A good partner will pick you up on down days and chew you out when you need it. What to look for in a partner? The best partner is consistent, responsible and positive. A negative approach can really scuttle the atmosphere so avoid anyone who always finds the bad side to everything.

A training partner does not necessarily have to be at the same level as you are – it is often best to pair up with someone more knowledgeable and glean from his or her years of experience. Working out with an experienced bodybuilder will knock years off your learning curve and greatly speed up your progress. If you prove to be a consistent partner and solid spotter to a bodybuilder in need, things should work out great for both of you.

The flip side of the coin is to train alone. The benefits here are deeper concentration on the muscles being worked – a real plus in musclebuilding – and the time between sets is not spent spotting your partner, but rather mentally preparing for your next set. Training alone also allows for more freedom in scheduling workout times (you don't have to wait for someone else to show up) and the flexibility to change arrangements whenever you want. Train alone or with someone else – both can be beneficial and either can work for you, depending upon your training temperament.

Working out with an experienced bodybuilder will knock years off your learning curve.

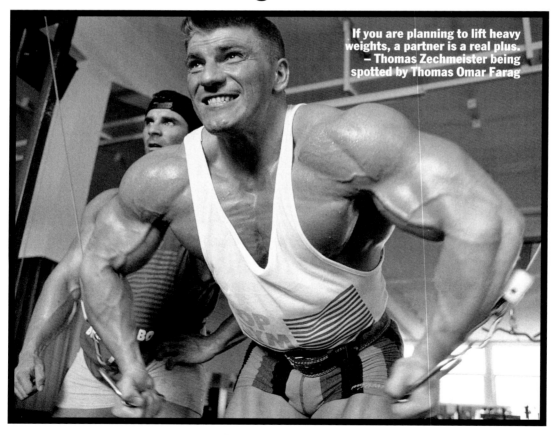

If you are planning to lift heavy weights, a partner is a real plus.
– Thomas Zechmeister being spotted by Thomas Omar Farag

Measure Up

Before you ever pick up your first weight, measure your body. Check out your weight and measure your arms, neck, chest, waist, thighs and calves. Also check your bodyfat level. Write everything down. Get a picture taken of yourself in a swimsuit. Store this data in a folder where you can use it to chart your progress as you move forward in changing the shape of your physique. Who knows, you may do so well in your training that you decide to enter one of those "before and after" transformation contests.

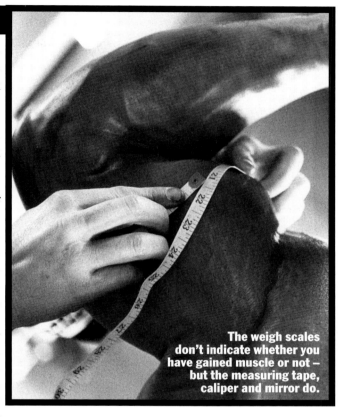

The weigh scales don't indicate whether you have gained muscle or not – but the measuring tape, caliper and mirror do.

The main reason for keeping track of this data is to realize the encouragement and even joy of seeing your body change from soft to solid, from rotund to muscular, or, if you are the anemic type, to see your physique finally move from skinny to muscular. You may *suspect* you are making progress, but the only way to know for sure is by mea-

Before you ever pick up your first weight, measure your body.

suring and accumulating data. The thinnest line is better than the thickest memory, so write it all down. No one but you needs to see it and it is valuable information to have at hand.

Measure the biceps in the flexed position, but measure the chest and legs in a relaxed position, each area at the peak of the muscle belly. Caliper and a tape will allow you to check bodyfat and waist girth. Naturally you want these calculations to start shrinking while the others grow. Don't be too alarmed if you hold even in bodyweight initially, even though you are working out hard. You've probably lost a few pounds of fat and gained a few pounds of muscle but the scales show the same overall weight. The scales don't really indicate whether the weight you have gained is muscle or not – but the measuring tape, caliper and mirror do. If you don't measure your physique and jot down your body statistics when you get started on a musclebuilding program, you miss a golden opportunity to observe changes from your baseline body condition – so measure *now*, before you get started.

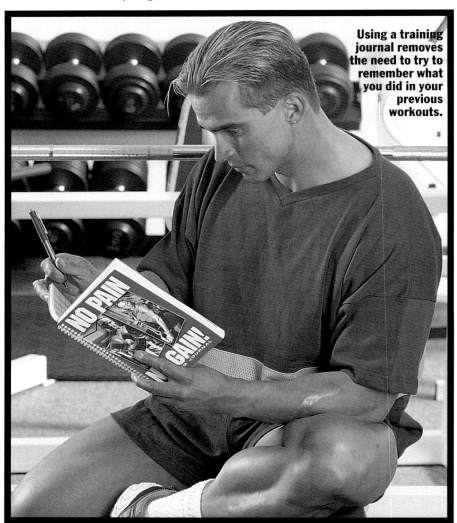

Using a training journal removes the need to try to remember what you did in your previous workouts.

Training Journal

Another key tool for tracking your physical progress is the journal. The training journal is a place where you can keep track of your body measurements, but it is designed more for tracking of the actual training sessions. Names of exercises used, poundages, number of repetitions and sets – all are noted in the training journal. Dates are also important to retain. You can use the training journal for more than just cold facts – you can write in your personal comments to help direct future training as well, explain why you missed a workout (got sick), etc. The more you use a training journal the more precise you can be in making adjustments and gathering insight on your progress. If progression has stopped and you need to change your routine, a training journal will make that obvious. A notebook of lined paper and a pen with an attachable clip will work fine, and won't cost you an arm and a leg either.

Example of a training journal entry:
December 15th
Squats – warm up, 200 x 10, 9, 7
Leg curls – 70 x 7, 10, 7
Lunges – 100 x 10, 10
Bent-over rows – 155 x 8, 7
Cable pulldowns – 135 x 7, 8, 6
Notes: Push myself harder on final squat set. Increase weight for lunge next workout. Add one more set of bent rows. Focus more on feeling the muscles work in the pulldown.

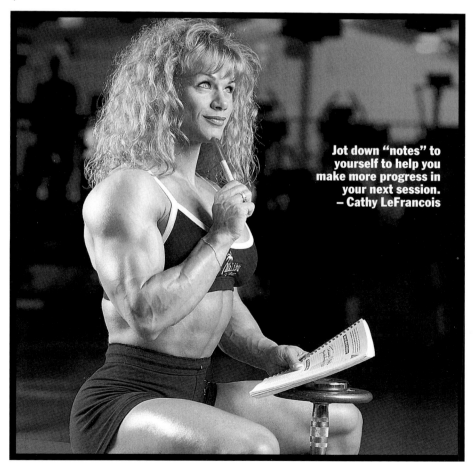

Jot down "notes" to yourself to help you make more progress in your next session.
– Cathy LeFrancois

Using a journal or chart removes the need to try to remember what you did. It effectively eliminates the guesswork and puts you in charge of where you are going. Write down information from the workout that will help you make more progress next time. Your notes can be as long or as short as you want, but make a habit of recording anything pertinent. Keep your old training journals. Stack them in storage or wherever, but make sure you can access them. They provide invaluable data for reconstructing previous routines. Here is another example of valuable training-journal information.

Example of training journal entry:

December 21st
Bench presses – warm up, 250 x 7, 5, 4
Incline bench presses – 200 x 10
Flyes – 45 x 8, 10
Barbell curls – 115 x 5, 7
Reverse curls – 55 x 9, 8

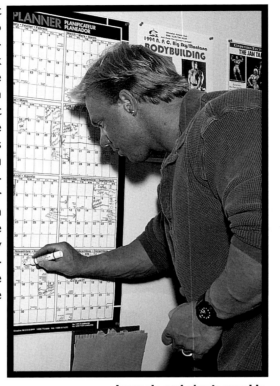

Journals and charts provide invaluable data for reconstructing previous routines. – Dave Fisher

Notes: Stay at current weight with bench press until I can get more reps. Add another set for incline bench. Go deeper in the flye. Add preacher curls to the biceps workout. Nutrition note: Buy more refuel carbo mix before next workout.

The training journal can be of great assistance in developing an understanding of your own unique body and its responses to training. Musclebuilding is a pursuit that is very empirical in nature, so the more you can document and categorize the events and your body's reactions the better.

When it comes to building the muscles up, many different vital aspects are involved. What I've mentioned so far is just the tip of the iceberg. However, before moving on, reread this chapter to make sure you have a good grasp on the concept. Start by building a good base and take the time on this important journey to make your beginning something special. Then you can move on to adding to that solid foundation.

Keys to a Firm Foundation

• Start simple with the squat and a few other basic exercises such as the overhead press, bench press, bent-over row, triceps pushdown and arm curls.
• Use a range of 8 to 12 reps for 2 sets during the first month, moving up to 3 sets thereafter.
• Apply the overload principle. Each set should include the final phase of 2 or 3 very difficult repetitions.
• Commit to safe training and focus on good form.
• Develop the habit of using a training journal for every workout.

Thoughts From the Pros on Building the Initial Foundation

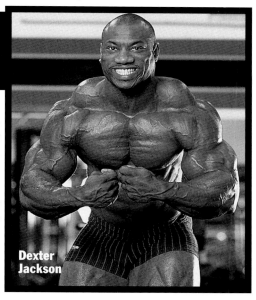

Dexter Jackson

Good form is important:
"Good form is always my number one priority. Since I use heavy weights, it's vital that I perform each rep carefully. Take the time to learn the proper mechanics of each movement — read books and magazines, and watch and talk to more experienced lifters in your gym. Even invest in a good personal trainer for a month or two to help take you to the next level."
– Dexter Jackson

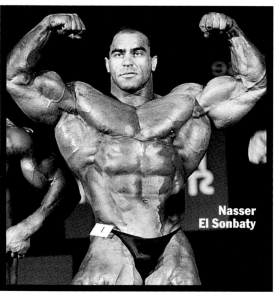

Nasser El Sonbaty

On the overload principle:
"To make a muscle grow, you've got to give it some kind of stimulus, some overload. When I started training I could bench press 130 pounds. Now I can bench press over 500 pounds ... It's simple, really: When you stress the muscle beyond what it's used to, it compensates and adapts to the stress by becoming stronger and larger." – Dorian Yates

More on muscle growth:
"To make a muscle grow you must force it to go beyond its capabilities. The most potent way to apply that force is to train to failure. Training to failure means exactly that ... the muscles are forced to grow stronger and bigger."
– Nasser El Sonbaty

2

WORKOUT STRATEGY –
SOFTWARE
FOR SUCCESS

Pressing and pulling the weights is how you change your body's shape and size. But the weightlifting is only the surface result of the real power a behind successful workout. The most important aspect of any musclebuilding program lies in an intangible element – workout strategy. You cannot see strategy as it is being concocted in someone's mind, but you can definitely see the results good strategy provides. Just as with software, the real value is in the design, application and feedback the program supplies. The uneducated often overlook this aspect and that is one of the reasons there is such a high failure rate when the novice becomes a gym member. Simply grasping the nearest tool and flailing away won't sculpt the body into an attractive shape. There has to be structure to the workout, and there must be order and purpose in that structure. A program will succeed in large part due to its design. Certainly intensity in application plays a large and important role, but without a solid and meaningful design, the outcome will be mediocre at best.

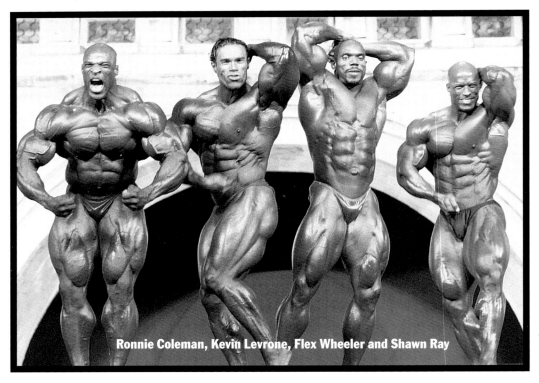

Ronnie Coleman, Kevin Levrone, Flex Wheeler and Shawn Ray

How can a beginner be expected to know how to come up with a successful workout strategy? It's not gonna happen – hence the high failure rate. Novices simply do not have the insight to design a great workout strategy from scratch. The few who have forged ahead have gone the trial and error route to rough out a strategy. But even they failed to *maximize* the muscularity of their physique. What has proved successful is the collective wisdom gathered from many who made the early journey into the frontier of the human skeletal muscle development. Fortunately these painstaking trial and error journeys have yielded a body of information that everyone who follows can use. To get off to a good start you don't have to reinvent the workout wheel – there are already several workable models.

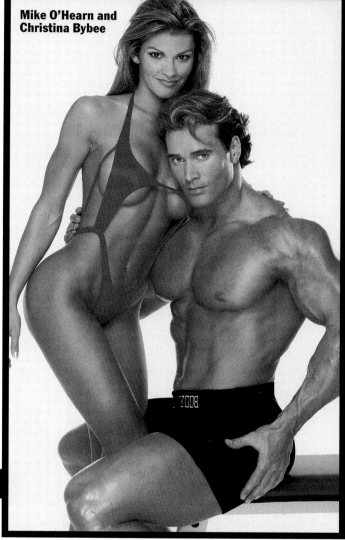

Mike O'Hearn and Christina Bybee

Two Tracks

There are two essential tracks to workout strategy. The first is best employed in the beginning stages of musclebuilding. This track involves using the workout strategy that others have found to be productive in stimulating their physiques to make muscle gains. Enough people have found common ground to make certain workout configurations a reliable approach to use. Those who have gone first have experimented and found what works and what does not work in stimulating the major muscle groups. Every body has a somewhat different response to a particular workout, but there is enough common ground in the human form in general to be able to classify certain routines as workable for large segments of the population. In the beginning stages of training it is very helpful to tap into this body of knowledge in order to make the quickest and surest muscle gains.

You can waste years of productive training if you start to experiment before you have a good grasp of the key principles and basic makeup of the central workout strategies.

Jay Cutler

The Next Level

Track two is considered the graduate school of musclebuilding, where new workout strategies and application methods are discovered. In fact, anyone who wants to maximize their own unique physique must first get to this point of development. You have to pay your dues on the basic well-known workout strategies before you move up to this level of intuitive training. Don't make the mistake of experimenting without first learning the theory behind musclebuilding. You can waste years of productive training if you start to experiment before you have a good grasp of the key principles and basic makeup of the central workout strategies. Some people make the mistake of experimenting too soon. Then, when they can't come up with anything that will make the muscles grow, they're discouraged. That's backwards.

Don't make this error. I have featured several approaches in the following pages to help you get a good start. Give yourself ample time to examine the different key strategies and how they work with your body before you branch out into something new. There is no law that says you have to start experimenting at a certain point. If a method is working well, by all means stay with it. Not until a workout strategy runs dry do you move on to something else. After trying several of these strategies, and milking them for all they're worth, then it's time to experiment. Use the knowledge of others as often as possible. Read all the bodybuilding books you can get your hands on. Subscribe to musclebuilding magazines. Get on the Internet and read what others find works for them. As you can now see, building muscle is as much or more a *mental journey* as it is a physical journey – so dig as deep as you can.

In track two you begin to learn all about your physique. Based upon what you have discovered to be your body's unique responses to the various training methods, you will start to put together some workable programs that produce results. At this point you are looking for that killer application, the workout that will take your physique to the next level of muscularity and beyond.

At what point do you switch from the track of using the workouts of others and move forward to create your own? There is no set time frame or date; however, you will suddenly realize one day that you are in fact making certain changes to your workout based on your personal insight and intuition. You want to get to this stage of *intuitive training*, where the gains really kick in. At this point you are no longer reliant upon the insight of others. You are coming up with your own. You must be willing to experiment, to be flexible, because in the advanced stages of training you will be aiming at a moving target. Your body will respond to certain workout configurations for only so long, then it will become familiar with the stimulus and cease to respond.

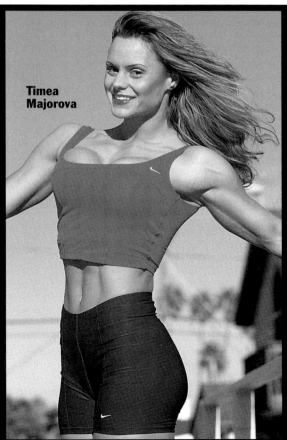

Timea Majorova

Shawn Ray points out in *Flex* magazine that the best way to ensure your body stays the same is to do the same thing all the time, and that, once you hit a plateau, you won't make progress unless you change your approach. Shawn makes the point that your *training* needs to evolve if you want your *body*

Make it your goal to get to the point of "intuitive training," where the gains really kick in for your unique physique.

to evolve to a new level of muscular development. You must rotate to something new to get it going again. Become your own training advisor. This does not mean you are beyond considering the insight and wisdom of others. Indeed, "*new*" discoveries are rarely made in this evolving science/art of musclebuilding (many are just improvements upon previous discoveries) and you can benefit from some of them (but not all). At this point you take responsibility for the strategic development of your physique instead of being spoonfed by a personal trainer or waiting for the next fad book. Not all musclebuilding fads work and by the time you've reached the intuitive stage you will be able to figure out quickly whether or not something

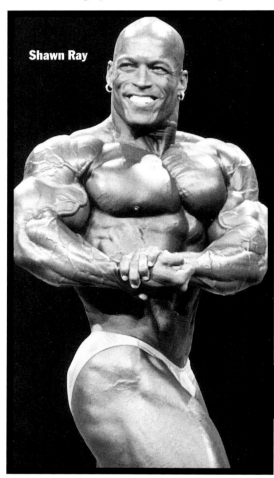

Shawn Ray

"Your training methods need to evolve if you want your body to follow suit." – Shawn Ray

will work for you. Again, a good goal for the long term is to reach this advanced stage. That is where you are headed. But first things first. The real work starts right now, at the *basic stages* where you look to others to provide you with some general road signs on the path to a more muscular physique.

Muscle-Growth Rhythm

When designing an overall workout strategy, the main concern is to structure the training in such a manner as to facilitate your efforts to integrate with (as well as prompt) the *muscle-growth rhythm* of your body. In training the human physique toward the desired goal of building muscle, there is a certain rhythm that must be acknowledged, anticipated and worked with. The equation in working the body is not a simple one-step "exercise input equals muscle output" formula. No, several powerful variables are involved. I'm warning you – ignore them at your own risk. If the body responded automatically by providing muscle in return for just any type of training input, everyone would be walking around sporting 26-inch arms. Guess what? We aren't. In fact, compared to the total number of bodybuilders out there, very few even have 20-inch arms. The same holds true

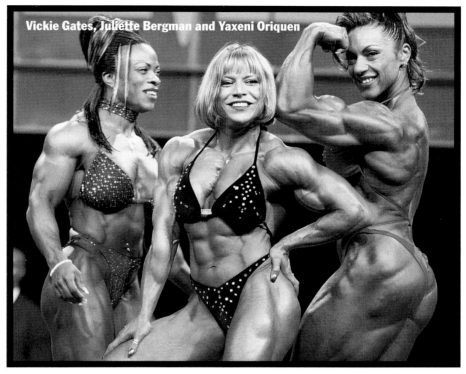

Vickie Gates, Juliette Bergman and Yaxeni Oriquen

for the rest of the body. You can't simply push some weights around and expect significant results. You won't maximize your physique – or even come close. The best place to start making progress is in working with, not against, the natural currents of the body. That means you must know your muscle-growth rhythm real well.

You must recognize the fact that actual muscle growth does not happen during training – it occurs after training, if enough rest and good nutrition is provided to the body.

The growth rhythm of the muscles is give and take, much like the tides of the sea. The body is given the stimulus for muscle growth by the tearing down of the muscles during a workout. The body will respond by growing more muscle – if it gets adequate rest. You must recognize the fact that actual muscle growth does not happen during training – it occurs after training, if enough rest and good nutrition is provided to the body. During training – specifically resistance training – the muscles being worked are actually torn down. If they receive significant (such as occurs with weightlifting) and constant tearing down without any down time between sessions to build back up, they will actually become smaller and weaker, not bigger and stronger. Some novices make the mistake of training the same

Deliberately allow time for muscle growth to occur.

bodypart day after day and wonder why they ache so much and have no gains in muscle size. The reason is, adequate rest has not been provided to the muscles.

Nutrition must also be factored in as another important aspect of musclebuilding or even more important. Consider the training progression of Brad Harris, who is fairly new to the musclebuilding scene. Brad has a sports background, a good work ethic, and pushes himself very hard in the gym. However, several months into his training he found himself exhausted by the end of his workouts, and stumbling through his final few sets. The remedy? More time off between sessions, and the addition of a sports drink during the workout and a nutrition bar afterward. Brad notes that this simple strategy is fantastic, saying, "The Gatorade has immensely improved my lifting. I get done faster. I also eat a power bar immediately after my workout. Then I stretch, of course." By adjusting to what his body needed, Brad got back on track to making muscle and strength gains.

Simply by getting in tune with your body's needs, you can make a real difference in the results you receive from your training. When designing your workout strategy, consider the way your body reacts. You can't just make something up out of the blue and expect it to produce maximum results. What you do must be grounded in the reality of your physique's response.

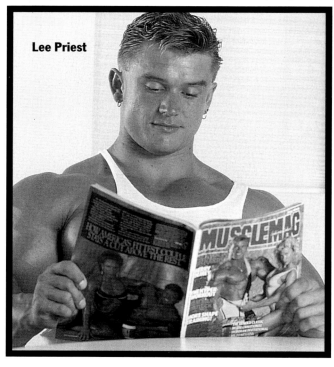

Lee Priest

Here is one major element of reality to recognize: Muscle-growth rhythm requires that your workout strategy allows a certain minimal time for rest between workouts. As pointed out, you do not work the same muscle group every day — that would be a recipe for certain disaster. Instead you deliberately allow time for the muscle to recover and grow. Training frequency varies from one person to the next. It also depends on the type of training. At the very least you must allow a full 48 hours of down time before you work the same muscle group again. Beyond this minimal requirement there is great variance. The extreme far end of the spectrum is championed by bodybuilders (such as the late Mike Mentzer) who believe one should allow for a couple of weeks or so between workouts for the same muscle group. Others find they can make gains with as little as 72 hours of rest and repair.

Expert guru, the late Vince Gironda once stated that a hard-worked muscle takes at least 72 hours to fully recuperate. Your goal is to find out what muscle-growth rhythm your own body does best with. Do your muscles bounce back quickly (say within 72 hours) or do they need a longer recuperation phase (maybe a week or so)? Start by experimenting with some of the workout systems recommended by the professionals. Remember to look for routines that the pros used in the beginning of their training, not their current system. A good initial approach to setting up a workout strategy is to go with a basic two-day split rotation, then eventually make adjustments.

Split Workouts

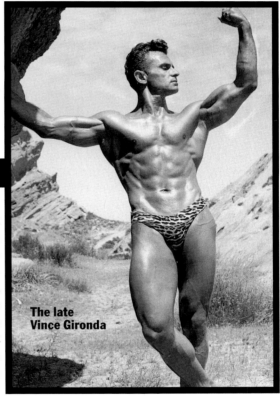

The late
Vince Gironda

In a split routine you don't train the whole body every workout. A split workout simply allows more time for concentration on specific muscle groups and gives you a chance to narrow your focus and really blast a region or two. Why not work the entire body in one shot? Of course the time element is important, but the energy and testosterone factors are crucial. Neither stay at high levels for a long period of time.

Energy in the form of transformed carbs (ATP and glycogen) is the best fuel source for the musclebuilding effort. However, the longer the workout continues, the lower the energy lamp burns. The same is true for the testosterone levels. Vince Gironda believed that a workout aimed at building the muscles up should last no longer than one hour, better still 45 minutes. Many professionals make it a point to not push past an hour, and the trend recently has been toward a shorter rather than longer training session. The longer you make the workout last, the lower your energy and testosterone levels drop. So does your concentration and desire. When your mind checks out of the gym, forget about it. Time to pack it in right then and there. The mind is the power

A split workout allows more time for concentration on specific muscle groups.

center for a dynamic workout and intensity is what sparks muscle growth. When the intensity burns out, it's time to head for the showers. The key is to get in a hard workout that hits the targeted muscles fully, then get out of the gym. The only real way to do this is to split the work into manageable sessions.

The most basic split is to divide the overall workout routine in half. However, you can take this approach a lot further. A routine can be double-split, triple-split, or more. Some bodybuilders designate a separate training session for each major muscle group. Others rotate muscle groups to get in at least two sessions per bodypart per week. In fact *hardcorebodybuilding.com* suggests the following, even for beginners:

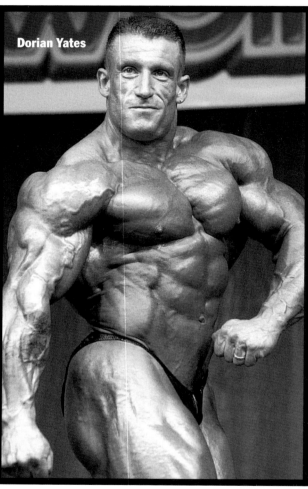

Dorian Yates

Monday – chest, tris and shoulders
Tuesday – back and bis
Wednesday – legs
Thursday – chest, tris and shoulders
Friday – back and bis
Saturday – legs
Sunday – rest

This workout can produce growth for a while. However, the drawback here is, you are almost always in the gym – there is only one day off per week. You can give this workout a go, but realize that there are many variations of the split workout system and none are set in stone. Frank Sepe has one of the hottest physiques around, and was lifting weights six days a week before backing off to his current rate of four times per week. Some bodybuilders train even more often than that on occasion. However, more common is the strategy of putting two or three muscle groups into one condensed workout.

Hardcore proponent Dorian Yates used a variety of split routines, one of which looked like this:

Day one – chest, back and shoulders
Day two – rest
Day three – legs, biceps and triceps

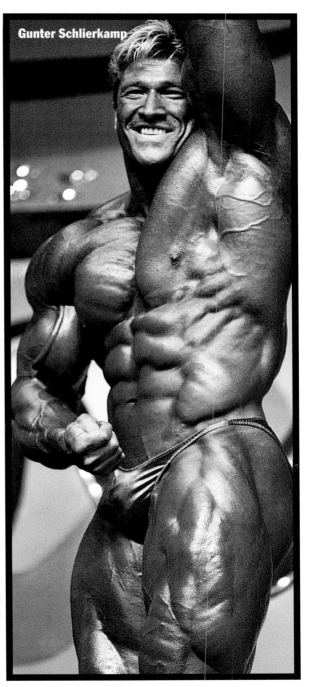

Gunter Schlierkamp

Yates grew on that split system. He noted that he liked it better than the three days on/one day off that most professionals opt for. Dorian does not stick with one split; he varies the routines as well. Another split he has used is:

Day one – delts, traps, triceps and abs
Day two– back and rear delts
Day three – rest
Day four – chest, biceps and abs
Day five – legs
Day six – rest

Dorian may change up the exercises within the rolling two-day split, but he likes to get that day of rest after two consecutive hardcore workouts and that is an approach you should also consider – at least one day of rest for every two days in the gym.

Gunter Schlierkamp also uses a two-day-on/one-day-off system, working a split that looks like this:

Day one – back and biceps
Day two – chest and triceps
Day three – rest
Day four – abs and legs
Day five – shoulders and calves
Day six – rest

Those two rest days are as important as the workouts. Some people need a day off training more often than others.

David Hawk, a professional bodybuilder currently trying to make a comeback, uses a traditional three-day-on/one-day-off split:

Day one – chest, triceps, shoulders and abs
Day two – back, biceps, traps, lower back/obliques and forearms
Day three – hamstrings, quads and calves
Day four – rest

David Hawk further mixes it up by doing one full session through the four-day rotation with heavier weights. Then the next time around he goes with lighter weights and some supersets.

Jay Cutler is one of bodybuilding's elite. His workout split once looked like this:

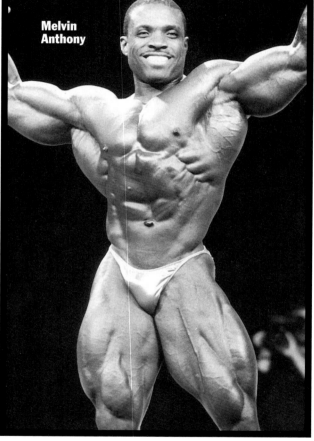

Melvin Anthony

Day one – chest, calves and cardio
Day two – back, abs and cardio
Day three – rest
Day four – shoulders, traps, calves and cardio
Day five – arms, abs and cardio
Day six – rest
Day seven – legs

Note that many of these routines are simply one variation used by that bodybuilder. All that may change a few months down the road. Shawn Ray tries to do something different every time he goes to the gym! NPC champion Melvin Anthony, a real animal in the gym, uses this workout split:

Day one – chest, shoulders and arms
Day two – back
Day three – legs
Day four – chest, shoulders and arms
Day five – back

Many bodybuilders allow more time for rest when they are not training for an upcoming contest. The stage of adding mass and allowing more rest is called *the off-season*. Even those who don't compete go through an off-season. Bodybuilder Dexter Jackson's off-season training split allows for more rest time. It looks like this:

Day one – chest, shoulders, biceps and calves
Day two – rest

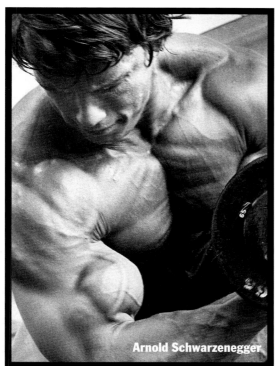

Arnold Schwarzenegger

Day three – quadriceps and hamstrings
Day four – rest
Day five – back, traps, triceps and calves
Day six – rest
Day seven – rest

Arnold Schwarzenegger suggests the following split for a person who has had some initial basic weight-training experience and is now ready to move up to a split routine:

Day one – legs, chest and abs
Day two – shoulders, back, arms, abs and calves
Day three – rest
Day four – legs, chest and abs
Day five – shoulders, back, arms, abs and calves
Day six – rest
Day seven – rest

Kevin Levrone is one of the hottest bodybuilders around, with a physique that features radical depth and full muscle bellies. He has been able to maintain an incredible body year after year. One of his workout splits looks like this:

Day one – chest, shoulders and triceps
Day two – back, biceps, hamstrings and calves
Day three – abs and quads
Day four – rest

Look over the various split routines of the top bodybuilders and you will notice a recurring theme. The muscles being worked are divided into groups – the chest, back, shoulders, traps, biceps, triceps, legs (quads, hamstrings and calves) and

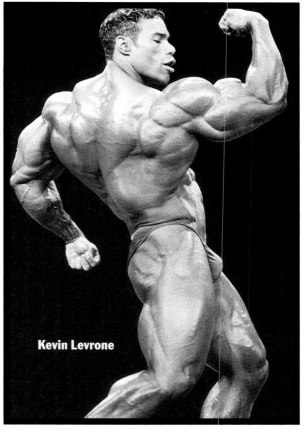

Kevin Levrone

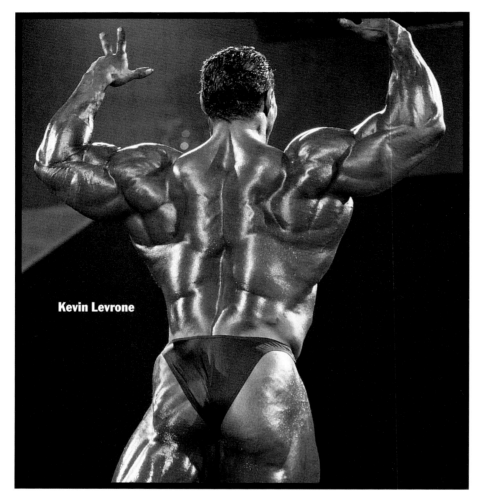

Kevin Levrone

abdominals. That is, exercises are not the focal feature of a workout – the muscles are. The workout is structured around the most important element, the major muscle groups. Bodybuilding is unique in this aspect. Powerlifting and Olympic lifting feature the exercises and the successful completion of a lift as the central aim. The relationship to muscles is of secondary concern. In bodybuilding the exercises play second fiddle to the muscles. To this end, almost every bodybuilder divides the body into muscle groups (then mixes these up – the split is rarely static). This chapter describes several different split routines, but these are just a sampling of the many types of splits possible.

Specific exercises work specific muscle groups. Curls, for instance, don't do much of anything for the quadriceps. The lateral raise does nothing for the calves. Certain exercises put the pressure on specific muscle groups. Knowing which exercises hit which muscles is handy (to say the least) when designing a training routine. Here is a list of which exercises target which major muscle groups:

Major Muscle Group	Exercises
Chest	Bench press, incline bench press, decline bench press, wide-grip dips, pec-dek machine, flyes, Incline flyes, incline dumbell twist, cable crossover, pushup, elevated pushup, seated machine bench press.
Shoulders	Overhead (military) press, behind-the-head press, dumbell press, lateral dumbell raise, front barbell raise, front dumbell raise, bent-over dumbell lateral raise, upright row, wide-grip upright row, seated machine press.
Trapezius & Neck	Traps: Shrugs (barbell and dumbell), standing machine shrugs, deadlift. For neck: neck raises (weight attached to harness), four-way neck machine, reverse neck raises, side neck raises from prone position.
Back	Chinups (front and rear), cable pulldown, bent-over row, machine pulldown (hammer style), T-bar row, dumbell row, deadlift, cable row (various styles), hyperextension (for lower back), good morning (for lower back).
Triceps	Close-grip dips, close-grip bench press, cable push-down, close-grip pushup, dumbell extension/ press, cable extension, lying and standing French press, Nautilus triceps machine.
Biceps & Brachialis	Barbell curls, dumbell curls, incline dumbell curls, close-grip barbell curls, close-grip chinups, biceps curl machine, EZ-bar curls, cable curls (various), 21s. For brachialis: reverse curls, Zottman curls, hammer curls, reverse preacher curls.
Abdominals	Crunches, leg lifts, half-range situps, hip rolls, bike crunches, abdominal vacuum, hanging leg raise, side bend (without weights), V-raise, bench leg lift, cable crunch, seated knee-up, hanging side knee raise.
Quadriceps	Squats, leg press, hack squat, sissy squat, front squat, leg extensions, lunges (barbell and dumbell), Smith-machine squats, Roman chair squats, non-lock squats.
Hamstrings	Leg curl, standing (one leg) leg curl, stiff-leg deadlift.
Calves	Standing calf raise, seated calf raise, calf press off leg press machine, one-leg calf raise with dumbell, donkey calf raise.
Forearms	Wrist curl, wrist roll-up, deadlift (matched grip), reverse curl, Zottman curl.

The general bodybuilding community have found these exercises to work best in targeting specific muscle groups. There are other exercises that will work your muscles, but these are simply the most commonly productive. If you find a movement that causes your muscles to grow like crazy, by all means use it. But stick with the tried and true in the beginning before branching out.

Muscle Rotation

A good place to start a simple split workout routine is to use a two-day-on/two-day-off training rotation. This schedule will give your body more time to become accustomed to the demands of the workout, and allow plenty of rest time so the muscles can grow back stronger. The second day of rest is justified because your input will be intense. The workout will be demanding – resistance training in general and weight training in specific taxes the body to the max. Go with a two-on/two-off split.

Two-On/Two-Off Split Workout
Day one – shoulders, chest and biceps
Day two – legs, back and triceps
Day three – rest
Day four – rest
Day five – shoulders, chest and biceps
Day six – legs, back and triceps
Day seven – rest
Day eight – rest
Continue to repeat this cycle.

Start the workout with a good full-body warmup. Three minutes on a treadmill and a few stretching motions will help. Then do some bodyweight only movements for the areas you will be training. Start the shoulders with a light overhead press. Then move on to 3 sets of dumbell presses. Do the dumbell presses from a seated position (this

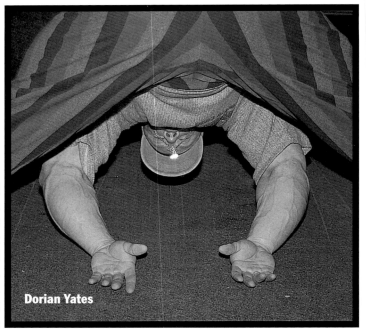

Dorian Yates

gives the best base). Allow yourself one to two minutes' rest between sets. Good rule of thumb: Do not start another set until you have caught your breath from the preceding set. Another rule is, rest longer between sets when your aim is mass and/or power; rest less when your aim is to get cut and trim. Work the shoulders hard with 3 sets of dumbell lateral raises. Aim for 10 repetitions of the presses and 12 of the lateral raises. For the lateral raises, hold the dumbell at the top of the movement (arms straight out) for a two-count, then slowly lower.

Choose this two-exercise combination and you will be in good company. It is the routine used by Ronnie Coleman when he started training – the dumbell press and dumbell lateral raise. He points out that the pressing movements are the "meat-packing side of the delt-building equation" due to the fact that they hit all three heads of the deltoids and really build thickness. The lateral raises whip up the width of the shoulders.

Chest Attack

Rest for a couple of minutes after your shoulder session, get a drink, then move on to chest. Your body will already be warmed up from

Good rule of thumb: Do not start another set until you have caught your breath from the preceding set.

the shoulder work but do warm up the chest before using heavier weights. After a warmup set of bench presses, move on to 3 sets of incline bench presses with a medium-width grip. Get a good deep drop, bringing the bar to the area where the neck and chest meet. Touch the top of the chest lightly, then press the bar up all the way. Try to get in 10 reps for each set. It is normal to lose

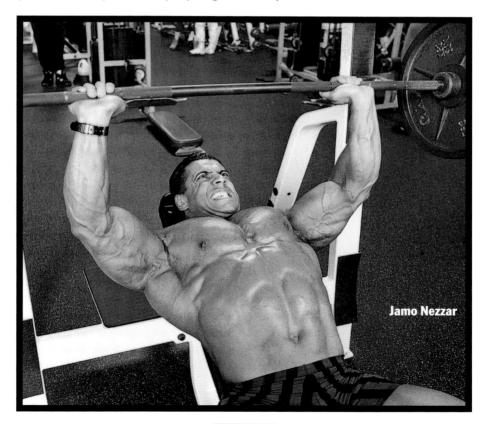

Jamo Nezzar

"Pressing movements are the meat-packing side of the delt-building equation." – Ronnie Coleman

a rep or 2 on the final set due to fatigue, but focus on keeping your form tight all the way through the entire movement. After the inclines, do 2 sets of the regular flat bench press with a higher repetition range. Get in 12 reps per set.

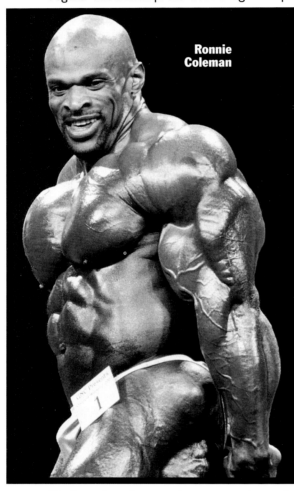

Ronnie Coleman

Finish the chest with a couple of sets of flyes. This movement is done as though you were hugging a very thick tree – get a good arc in the motion, and do not keep your arms straight. Bend your elbows slightly to release some of the pressure from the joints. Flyes work the chest in a very different manner than does the bench press, enabling you to tax the massive pec region with a deeper stretch. Go light with this movement initially, both in distance and weight. Then start pushing up the poundage and extending down toward the floor. Stop the flye just short of touching the dumbells together at the top of the movement. Do not lock out. Always move at a moderate pace to prevent injury. Go with a higher range of 12 reps for this movement also.

Rest for a few more minutes before wrapping up this session with almost everyone's favorite, the biceps. There is a strategy being employed here. It is easier to finish up a tough workout with a favorite exercise than with a non-favorite. Placing a favorite muscle group at the end also ensures that you finish as strong as you start, and stay interested to the end.

Another training principle employed in this particular workout strategy is the larger-to-smaller musclebuilding scheme. In general, it is best to work on the larger muscles first, then move to the smaller muscle group. You can alternate this approach now and then, but the larger-to-smaller progression is generally most productive.

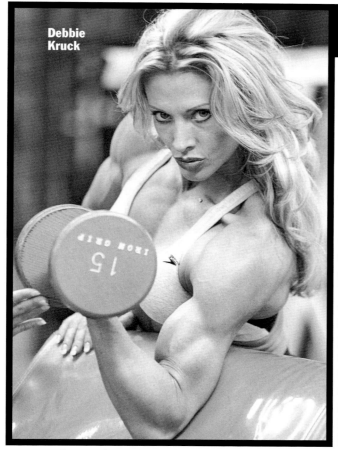

Debbie
Kruck

Ultimate Biceps-Builder

Start the last segment of the workout with the preacher curl, probably the ultimate biceps-building movement because it effectively elimnates all cheating action. You can't use momentum when you have the preacher bench pressing against the back of your arm and your upper body is draped at such an angle that any outside advantage is eliminated. There is no body boost when you use the preacher bench. The aim of the preacher bench is to take away any advantage the body may have outside the simple motion of the biceps. This makes it more difficult to hoist the weights, but the benefit is the biceps are the only muscle working. And in turn, that muscle will grow – radically.

The preacher curl forces *purity* into the motion, and teaches you how to isolate the biceps. One of the best decisions a novice can make is to use the preacher bench to learn how to focus on the biceps. Knowledge of the specific arc and pressure necessary for only biceps involvement can be translated to other biceps movements to ensure maximum stimulation from them as well.

The preacher curl forces purity into the motion, and teaches you how to isolate the biceps.

Before getting started, warm up the biceps with a set of regular curls for 10 to 12 repetitions. Then move on to the challenging preacher curl. When using the preacher bench, move at a moderate speed, particularly in the lowering of the bar to the extreme bottom position. Both your biceps muscles and your elbow joints are vulnerable at this point, so don't move quickly. Curl the weight back up, and stop at the point where the bar is just over the elbows. By stopping here you keep constant tension on the biceps – and constant tension equals quicker growth. If you go beyond this point you allow the tension to come off the biceps and they rest, which is not good for growth. Keep that tension on the biceps throughout the movement. Sure, it hurts more this way, and forces deeper concentration, but that is part of the formula for growth.

Rest is great on your days off; rest in the middle of an exercise will negate all your hard work.

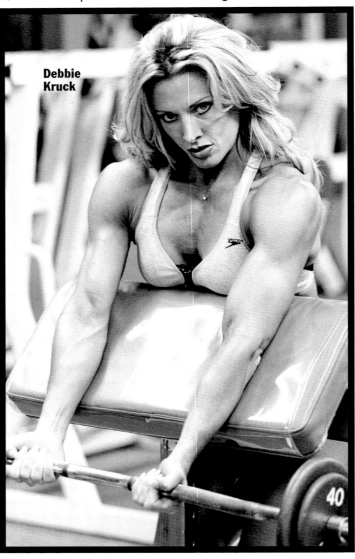

Debbie Kruck

Do 10 reps for 3 sets of preacher curls. Concentrate heavily on the action throughout the full motion. Squeeze the biceps muscle at the top, and feel the full extension in the down stroke. Shake and stretch the biceps, then move on to the final exercise of the first split workout, incline dumbell curls (alternated). The incline angle allows for a nice, deep stretch of the biceps. When you incline your body you give the biceps a longer arc than in the standing position. This longer arc stretches the biceps further throughout the working range – a good process for muscle growth. For bringing the most concentration to bear on the biceps, curl the dumbells one arm at a time (alternately, one arm then the other). Let the non-working arm hang down, dumbell in hand, with a slight tension while the other arm works. Do 3 sets of 8 repetitions of this excellent exercise.

The first workout of the two-part split is complete – but allow yourself a couple of minutes of flexing and stretching the physique before you walk out the door. Focus primarily on stretching the specific muscle groups that have just been worked. Then make it a point to get a good night's sleep and some tasty nutrition so that you can recover. That way the next workout will also be productive.

Initial Split Workout – Session I

Exercise	Sets	Repetitions
Barbell presses: warmup	1	10-12
Seated dumbell presses	3	10
Dumbell lateral raises	3	12
Bench presses: warmup	1	10-12
Incline bench presses	3	10
Bench presses	2	12
Flyes	2	12
Barbell curls: warmup	1	10-12
Barbell preacher curls	3	10
Incline dumbell curls, alternated	2	8

In addition to the light warmup sets, this routine consists of 6 sets for the shoulders, 7 for the chest, and 5 sets for the biceps – a total of 18 sets. Trainers typically place more of a workload (in terms of both weight and sets) on the larger muscle groups and less load on the smaller groups – hence the 5 sets for the biceps. Use enough weight on each exercise so that the final 2 or 3 repetitions are hard to do and make you push past the pain barrier.

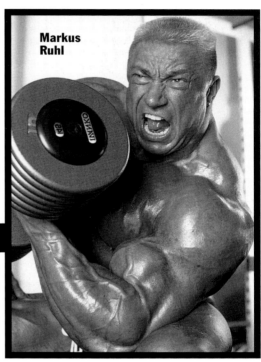

Markus Ruhl

Pain Barrier

The pain barrier is an unseen point in this intangible aspect, analogous to the wall in running, when you bump up against something not visible but very real. The muscles catch on fire and it becomes hard to complete the rep. *SpanerFitness* notes:

"When exercising, waste products and lactic acid are produced in the muscle cell. This condition is commonly referred to as 'the pump,' and it eventually leads to muscular failure. The amount of lactic acid in the muscle tissue is proportionate to the amount of cortisol released into the muscle tissue. It is the cortisol that actually tears down muscle tissue in the human body. Following this occurrence, the body will adapt by repairing the muscle tissue to its previous state and then growing a slightly greater quantity of muscle tissue than the body had previous to the workout."

The point in the set at which the muscles begin to fail due to lactic acid and waste accumulation and other related factors is what causes the pain – the accumulation builds up after several repetitions. Many people quit at this point, not wanting to have to handle the weight load and the pain it now brings. This is a mistake. Most of the growth stimulation comes beyond the pain barrier. The key to making good gains in muscle size and strength is to get *beyond the pain barrier*. There is no erasing the pain – the only way to handle it is with mental toughness. Top bodybuilders have learned how to accept and deal with the pain and push beyond the barrier to get in the extra few reps that give the growth. These final 2 or 3 repetitions are golden. This is where most of the gains made by the muscles occur. In fact the first several repe-

> *The key to making good gains in muscle size and strength is to get beyond the pain barrier. The final 2-3 reps beyond the pain barrier are "golden." They produce most of the muscle gains.*

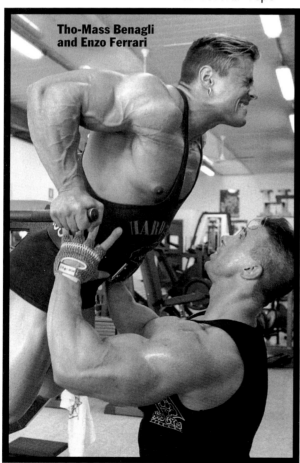

Tho-Mass Benagli and Enzo Ferrari

titions serve to set up the final few reps when the muscles are given the stimulus to grow. If you make it a practice to quit at the onset of the pain, you are basically limiting your body growth into a rut. Go through the pain barrier. Beyond the pain barrier lies the real growth zone. Muscles don't get bigger and stronger voluntarily – they need a good reason to do so. Busting past the pain barrier is that reason. The pain barrier is a reality and a part of every productive weight-training session. If you can't handle the pain, you won't get the gains. It's that simple. All of the top bodybuilders are very tough mentally and much of that strength comes from having to face and push past the pain barrier every time they train.

Knowing the pain barrier exists and that you have to beat it is the first step in moving toward real muscularity. The most impor-

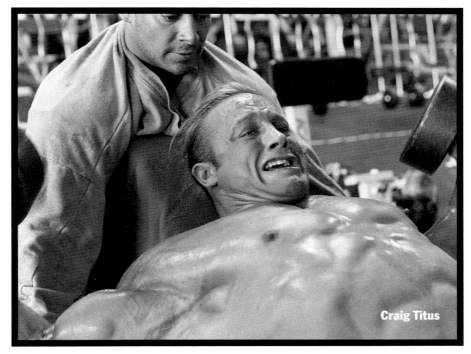

Craig Titus

If you can't handle the pain, you won't get the gains. It's that simple.

tant step, however, is application – doing it in the gym. That is where your willpower and desire to improve your body come to the forefront. If you want something bad enough, you can get it. Go beyond the pain barrier to those impressive gains that this type of training yields.

Session 2

The second workout of the split involves large muscle groups, the legs and the back, and the smaller muscle group, the triceps. Warm the entire body up. Then start the workout with legs. Go through the squatting motion without weights to unlock the knees. Move to a light squat for 10 to 12 repetitions. Keep the head up, shoulders parallel with the floor. Practice good form in the warmup set so that it becomes automatic when you move on to the heavier stuff. Add weight to the bar and start squatting. Do 2 sets of 12 reps. Go down until the thighs are parallel with the floor, then explode back up. Use a weight that makes you work. The squat is very taxing so do only 2 sets at this point. After the last set of squats, stretch the legs – particularly the quads.

Move on to the hamstrings and do 3 sets of leg curls. Keep your hips tucked tight against the bench throughout the movement. If you raise your hips

The calves are a dense muscle group that typically need a lot of stimulation to respond. Don't hesitate to blast them.

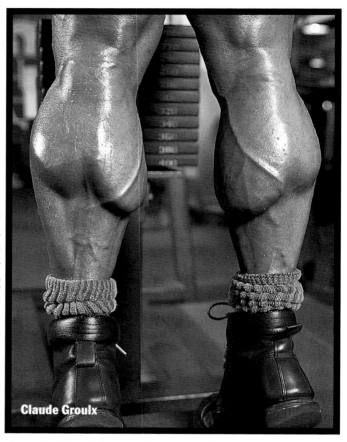

Claude Groulx

you take some of the emphasis away from the hamstrings and open the door to a possible injury. Move at a moderate to slow speed and don't linger at the top or bottom position. Keep that tension strong on the hamstrings at all points. When finished, stretch the hamstrings out nicely. Flex them as well. Learn how this unique muscle feels in action so you can do hamstrings work more intelligently.

Finish off the legs with 3 strong sets of raises on the standing calf machine. Warm up the calves first with some deep stretching off the platform, then duck under the pads and get started with the real weight. Go all the way down and all the way up. You want to get a really deep burn in the calves as they are a dense muscle and need powerful stimulation to grow.

Back Blast

Rest a few minutes, then move on to training the back and traps. Begin with 3 sets of bent-over rows. Load the bar and crank out 8 repetitions per set. After the rowing go to the chinning bar. The chinup, particularly the wide-grip chinup, greatly promotes wide back muscularity. Do 3 sets of this great exercise for as many repetitions as possible. Go all the way down and go up far enough to get your chin over the bar.

"Back injuries are sometimes caused by a strength imbalance between the lower back and abdominals, so it's important to train your abs frequently."
– Carol Ann Weber

Now load up a barbell for shrugs. This move is *primal* in nature — a basic power movement. Nasser El Sonbaty describes the motion: "Holding the barbell at thigh level with palms facing inward, shrug the shoulders and raise the bar as high as possible based on your range of motion. He also notes you should select a weight that will force you to failure on the final rep of each set. Multi-Mr. Olympia Ronnie Coleman, likes to use a heavy weight in a straight-up-and-down shrugging motion, focus on keeping the arms straight and holding the peak contraction. For this routine do 2 sets of 8 to 10 repetitions. Catch your breath, take a few swigs of water, and gear up to switch over to triceps.

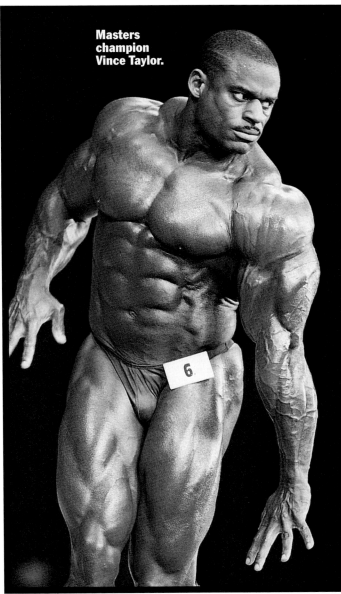

Masters
champion
Vince Taylor.

6

Terrific Triceps

The final muscle group targeted in this workout is the triceps. Always warm up well before starting, as training the triceps tends to aggravate the elbow area if they are not sufficiently warmed up before you start. Again, as with session one, we go from larger muscle groups to smaller, the triceps being the final muscle group in the routine.

The first exercise is the lying French press. This movement gives the cable pushdown a close run for being the most commonly used triceps exercise by top bodybuilders. In fact the lying French press may prove to be the number one triceps-training movement ever. The lying French press was a favorite of both Arnold Schwarzenegger and Dorian Yates. Between them they hold 13 Mr. Olympia titles. Considering that, you might want to make the lying French press your favorite as well. This move is also frequently used by almost all other top stars in their routines. It is a good exercise to consistently include in any triceps workout.

Keep your elbows in tight during the lying French press – no flaring. This rule holds true for most triceps motions.

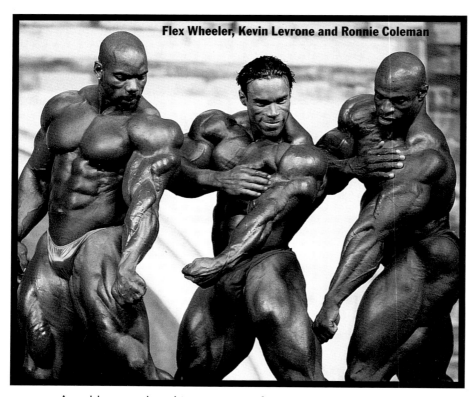

Flex Wheeler, Kevin Levrone and Ronnie Coleman

Arnold notes that this exercise is fantastic because it works all three heads of the triceps (whereas many others, such as the cable pushdown, don't). Arnold states the importance of keeping the arms angled at roughly just below 45 degrees to the body throughout the movement, lying prone on a bench. A barbell is held overhead (or dumbells) and lowered to either the forehead or beyond. Some bodybuilders call this movement the "skullcrusher" due to the bar hanging right above the forehead in the down position. If you choose to bring the bar down farther, you can lean your head off the back of the bench and get a deeper stretch in the triceps. Don't allow the elbows to drift out to the sides during the French press (or any other triceps work for that matter).

Nothing makes bodybuilding trainer Ollie McClay roar with disapproval quicker than seeing a trainee flare out the elbows during the lying French press. Instead of falling for this common mechanical mistake, deliberately keep your elbows tucked in tight at all times. Move slowly on this one, especially since the down stroke involves holding the bar right above your brain. The upstroke of the move should finish just short of 45 degrees so that the muscles are under constant tension. Do 10 repetitions in good form, allowing the hands to move the bar while the upper arm remains rigid. Get in 4 sets of this musclebuilder.

Wrap up the triceps with 2 sets of reverse dips. This move is done by placing your feet on a bench and your hands on another bench positioned behind you. Use a narrow hand placement, only a few inches apart. Dip down as far as possible, then press your body back upward to full arm extension. Once you have done this movement a few times, make it more challenging. Place a weight plate on your lap. The added resistance will make your triceps have to work harder – and they will grow more in return. Go for as many reps as you can possibly attain.

At the end of your session give yourself a brief cooldown period and stretch out the muscle groups you have just trained.

Initial Split Workout – Session 2

Exercise	Sets	Repetitions
Squats: warmup	1	10-12
Squats	2	12
Leg curls	3	12
Standing calf raises	3	10-12
Bent-over rows	3	8
Chinups	3	as many as possible
Barbell shrugs	2	8-10
Lying French presses	4	10
Reverse dips	2	as many as possible

This routine has a few more sets than does the first part of the split. However, it has fewer sets devoted to the upper body (only 14 as compared to 18 on the earlier routine). Mentally you can segment this session into two parts – hit the legs hard, rest a bit, then go to work on the upper body.

Time Off

Now comes the enjoyable part – taking a couple of days off. Literally take a few days off – don't be running around pushing your body to the limit in some other pursuit. People have a hard time gearing down, but that is what you need to do to enable your muscles to grow. After you've done both parts of the split routine (days one and two), you will definitely need to allow yourself a few days' rest. Do a couple of sets of ab work on your days off, if you want, but nothing more. If you have pushed your physique hard; if you have been working out beyond the pain barrier; if you have been moving heavy weights … you need rest. Your body will soon tell you so – it will ache! One good way to find out if you are hitting the muscles you intend to in training is to simply observe where you ache in the off days. You will ache. Rest is required. What you want to do now is maximize the time for anabolism.

Anabolism & Catabolism

When you lift weights you tear down the muscle tissue. Your body is forced into a catabolic state where, as noted previously, cortisol is released into the muscle tissue. It is the cortisol that actually tears down muscle tissue in the human body. Following this occurrence, the body will adapt by repairing the muscle tissue to its previous state and then growing a slightly greater quantity of tissue than the body had previous to the workout."

The body adapts to the impact of the workout by repairing itself and growing stronger – but only if it is given a good amount of rest and sound nutrition. To make good gains, don't underestimate the importance of rest, recovery and nutrition.

Consider the theory of Han Selye's General Adaptation Syndrome, which can be summed up as follows:

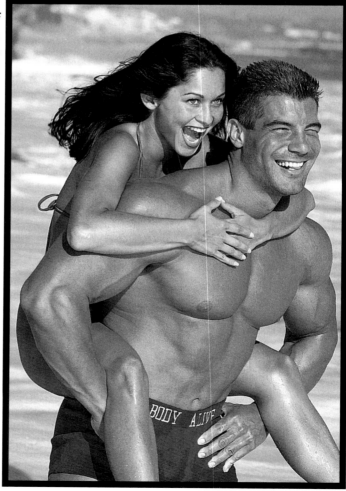

"In order to improve, you must balance challenge with recover." If you disregard this crucial theory you will hinder your progress. It is foolish to push the body to the extremes that weight training requires on a constant basis without planning for and allowing adequate recuperation and nutrition. The National Strength and Conditioning Association's guidelines for resistance training state that "the toleration and recovery from resistance-exercise stress is a crucial factor that must be monitored carefully in every resistance-training program."

What if you fail to observe Selye's theory and do not balance the stress of the workout with adequate recovery? The body will then slip into a degenerative state and not make it back again before your next workout. The breakdown of muscle tissue that occurs during exercise is not fully addressed. Energy has been depleted and tissue damage has taken place. The extreme demands of lifting heavy metal workout after workout can cause a deeper catabolism than a mild routine would. The split-workout system puts the body under strong stress two days in a row. At that point getting plenty of rest is job one. The body needs down time to make repairs, and you must facilitate that requirement with sleep and solid nutrition. This is the anabolic state.

If you ignore the importance of rest and repair, your muscles are doomed to minimal growth.

Energy is now being replenished and tissue repaired. Note that this anabolic state does not occur during the workout but rather *during rest* (especially during sleep), and is fueled by good nutrients. Time off is the anabolic time. Make sure you get adequate rest and good nutrition at this point. That does not necessarily happen automatically. The demands of daily living (busy work schedule, late night on the town, etc.) can interfere and prevent maximum recuperation from taking place. However, your goal is to rebuild the muscle tissue that was damaged during the intense exercise sessions. That is the objective for the two days off before your next workout. When you use resistance training as part of your routine (particularly weight training), your

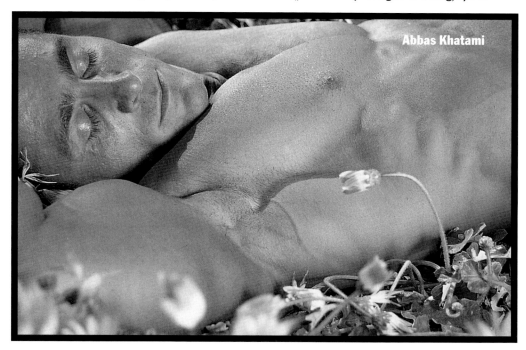

Abbas Khatami

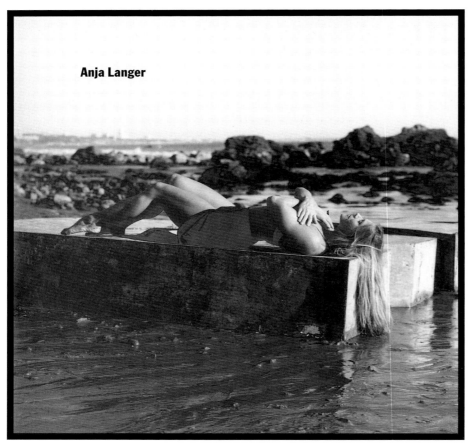

Anja Langer

recovery plan must have two principal aspects. Before the next session you must replace the energy and nutrients burned off during the workout and provide a bit extra to accommodate new growth.

To build muscle you need the power to push the body to a new level of physical development. This will require the building up of strength and size. The growth factor is a prime aspect as it involves more than mere replenishment – it necessitates more than just returning to the status quo and expecting a stride toward the next level – more muscle growth.

Being able to top the next workout level is important but even that is not enough. You want muscle growth – and for that your recovery from the last workout must *exceed* 100 percent (the growth factor makes up the additional percentage). Muscles don't grow in a vacuum – they need nutrition and rest to sprout up. Anabolic recovery is of prime importance for anyone seeking to increase the muscularity of the body itself, as tough workout sessions thrive on a full tank. In the following chapter the focus will turn to the nutritional aspect and how to maximize your strategy. At this point you must realize you will be approaching this next workout sequence stronger and with slightly bigger muscles than when you started out.

More Workout Strategy

You can train two days on/two days off for the next three months, increasing the amount of weight you use each time you are able to top the suggested repetition range. Add roughly 10 percent of the poundage you have been using and work back up to the suggested number of repetitions. You are using 60 pounds in the preacher curl, for example, and for the last couple of workouts you have been able to do your 10 reps fairly easily (the pain barrier is now hitting at about rep 10 or 11 instead of 6 or 7). You can then add five more pounds to the bar and start working with this new heavier load. The increase will most likely cause your rep range to drop and the pain barrier will be lower as well. Hit the workouts hard again, get adequate rest and nutrition, and over the next few weeks the reps will once again become easy as the muscles grow.

Exercise & Muscle Group Order

There is no law that says certain exercises must be done in a specific order. The general principle is to target the larger muscle groups first, the smaller groups second. However, even this rule of thumb can be violated on occasion and still yield good results. Now is the time to experiment with the order in which you do the different exercises. Don't always start with the same muscle group. Shawn Ray changes his exercise order for every major muscle group. He will even be so bold as to put squats at the end of a leg workout – that is a real challenge.

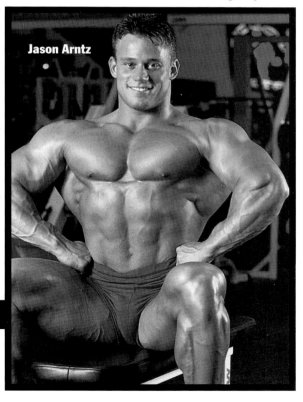

Jason Arntz

One approach worth mentioning is to work your weak areas first. This strategy is called prioritization. You put priority on the areas you want to bring up to speed. If your triceps are a weak link, you want to move them up to the top of the list. Work them first so they receive the most training energy and your best concentration.

Set Strategy

There are still more elements involved in designing a comprehensive workout strategy than just the number of repetitions and sets, exercises and muscle group priori-tation. One training technique employed by intermediate to advanced body-builders is called *supersetting* – performing two sets without resting between exercises. There are several ways to employ this interesting and challenging stimulation strategy:

Superset = 2 nonstop sets
Triset = 3 nonstop sets
Giant set = 4 nonstop sets

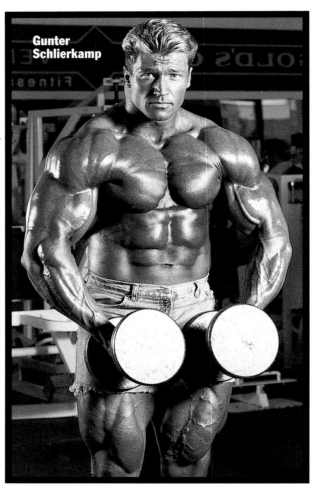

Gunter Schlierkamp

Supersets allow the workout to be less time-consuming, and also enhance a quicker pump, the rush of blood into the area being worked as waste is removed. The pump makes the muscles expand rapidly and notice-ably. Any exercise can bring about a pump; the superset will bring it about quicker. Furthermore, the superset is often used on opposing muscle groups in the same body region. By supersetting triceps with biceps an enor-mous pump can be realized, pushing the arms to new levels. Trisets, three nonstop sets, are often used on the same muscle to blast the muscle group from several angles and with different types of stimulation. Finally, giant sets are four sets done nonstop.

These training tricks are used on occasion by advanced athletes to squeeze out more growth. However, it is not a good idea to use the multiset approach all the time. One drawback is a lower level of concentration and effort in the final sets. Of all multiset training approaches, the superset is most frequently used, the most productive, and the one you can experiment with from time to time. Simply set up two exercises and do a set of each without resting between exercises. Then take a short rest and do the second superset. You might do one set of barbell curls and immediately move to a set of cable curls, for example.

Superset ...	Barbell curls	2 sets, 10 reps
with ...	Cable curls	2 sets, 8 reps

Supersets work well for a certain length of time, then you can go back to single-set workout approach. Vary the inclusion of supersets; when a routine gets *too routine*, bring supersets into play and get the blood really pumping again.

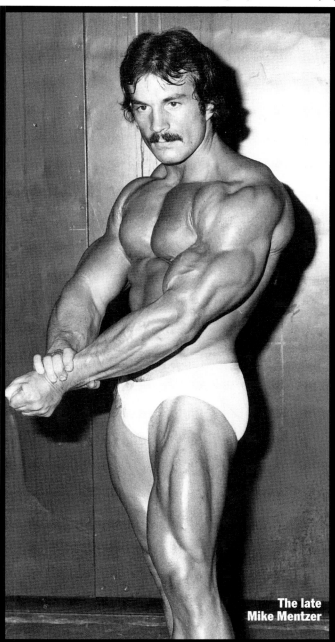

The late
Mike Mentzer

The number of sets you do can also be varied. You may want to choose a single exercise and do half a dozen sets. Vince Gironda championed his famous 8 sets of 8. Some shock routines go as high as 10 sets (this approach is only used briefly to shock the muscles). Recently under the onslaught of the heavy-duty movement the number of sets used by many bodybuilders has dropped back to 1 to 3 per exercise. However, some bodybuilders still do multiple sets per exercise and body-part, and grow well on the multiset strategy. Recent research noted in strength and conditioning journals indicates that multiset training is better for strength gains.

In the early days of bodybuilding, only a few sets were done per exercise. Then bodybuilders such as Leroy Colbert discovered that performing many sets could increase muscle growth. When Colbert went from a couple of sets per exercise up to 6 sets he experienced noticeable growth. On the flip side, both Dorian Yates and the late Mike Mentzer were able to grow more the opposite way, eliminating the high-set workout in place of just 1 or 2 very hardcore sets per exercise. Your body may respond better to more sets per exercise, or less. The only way you will every know is to try both ways, give each method time to do its stuff, and observe which approach brings about the best muscle gains.

Pyramid Scheme

A favorite of many bodybuilders, the pyramid technique involves the use of heavier weights and fewer sets in an ascending order of completion. Lou Ferrigno gave an example of pyramiding for the bench press in one of his books:

Bench Press
Set of 135 pounds for 12 repetitions
Set of 205 pounds for 10 repetitions
Set of 255 pounds for 8 repetitions
Set of 305 pounds for 6 repetitions
Set of 340 pounds for 4 repetitions
Set of 360 pounds for 2 repetitions

Of course you may not be able to handle as much weight as Lou, but this example provides a good overview of the way this technique works. He points out that pyramiding allows you to warm up thoroughly, do some midrange reps for shape and muscle quality, and then get in some low-rep sets for mass and power. You should definitely try the pyramid approach to see if it will spark some growth for your physique.

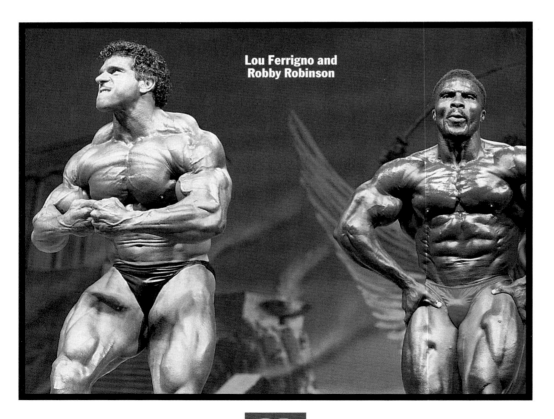

Lou Ferrigno and
Robby Robinson

Training Cycles

Cycling the training program is one of the most prevalent methods of controlling physical development. As has been hammered home throughout this chapter, it is not wise to use the exact same workout all the time. You do need to stick with the same routine for a certain period of time to observe strength and muscle changes and growth patterns (or the lack thereof) – but don't use the same old stuff forever. Your muscle gains will stop dead in their tracks if you do. The answer is to cycle your training.

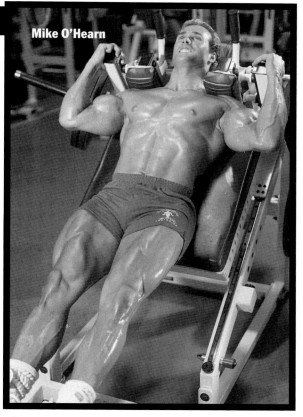

Mike O'Hearn

A training cycle is the period of time when you employ a certain workout routine. It is not designed to last forever; it has a specific beginning and end point. Professional bodybuilders are known to have three distinct training phases: off-season, contest preparation, and precontest. The off-season is when the focus centers on adding new muscle size and letting the body get more rest. Contest preparation is more intense and precontest training is the most intense of all. There are many variations of cycles, and you can make up your own entirely new cycle if you wish. Training cycles are sometimes grouped by the length of the cycle.

A training cycle is the period of time when you employ a certain workout routine. It is not designed to last forever; it has a specific beginning and end.

Another closely related term is *periodization*, which refers to the way training is broken down into discreet time periods called macrocycles, mesocycles and microcycles. Macro, of course, is the longest cycle and micro shortest. Sometimes there are even cycles within cycles. A cycle is a period of time when a specific goal is aimed for with a certain type of training. The workouts within that cycle may stay the same for the duration of the cycle, or they may change (a macrocycle may be made up of several microcycles).

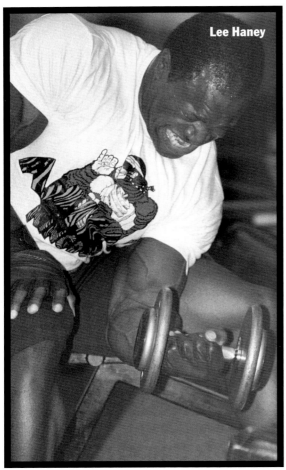

Lee Haney

If you want to pack on body mass, go on a cycle where all training strategies as well as nutrition are definitely geared toward cranking up the mass. Or you may want to trim down and go on a cycle that facilitates more fat loss than normal. A cycle can be set up for either end of the spectrum, or a hundred points in between. You can peruse the training of the stars to get some idea of the vast array of cycles available and possibly find something to use. As you become more comfortable with your own training judgement, you can then put together your personal cycle.

Start off with a definite goal — more muscle size, or to build up a certain area ... or maybe you even want to compete. Define the beginning and end of the time frame. Set up the split rotation with the exercises, sets and repetition ranges. Then start working your routine. You may find you need to make adjustments to maximize your workouts. Write them down. The next cycle will be even better. Soon you will be able to design productive workout cycles, not only for yourself but for others as well.

Intensity

The motor that powers any workout strategy to success is another intangible — *intensity*. To make positive changes to your physique you need to employ training intensity. If there is one common pole that draws all successful bodybuilders, it is intensity. Intensity is the intangible element that molds the metal of the weights into muscles as strong as metal. Incorporate intensity into every workout. That means no playing around or letting your mind drift. If you want to succeed in shaping a new physique, you will need to be all business in the gym. Once you step through the doors of the gym, it's all-out warfare for mastery of your body. Don't let mediocrity slow you down. Work the iron until you hurt. Keep the session fairly brief but go all out for the entire time you are there. Motivation and concentration will bring about the required level of intensity necessary to make impressive muscles.

Intensity is the intangible substance that molds the metal of the weights into the muscles that are strong as metal.

Strategy is the key to your success. A good workout strategy that intelligently incorporates all the variables – exercises, sets, rep range, breaking past the pain barrier, routine split by muscle group, cycled workouts, adequate rest and nutrition, one that is applied with *intensity* – will force the body to give you what you want ... more muscularity.

• Start your training strategy by absorbing all the information on musclebuilding you can from as many sources as possible. Piggy-back on the insight of others and use proven routines to get a quick and successful start. Rely on tried and true workout strategies for a solid foundation.
• Once you have learned the basics and tried several training strategies, you begin to observe your body's unique responses. Then and only then should you move up to the next level, where you can start to experiment and build your own workout strategies to become master of your own physique.

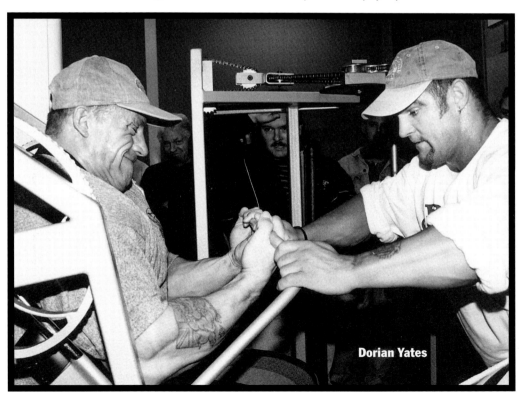

Dorian Yates

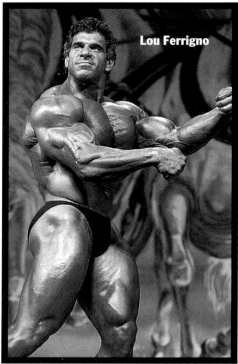

Lou Ferrigno

Thoughts From the Pros on Workout Strategy

Not every routine works the same for everyone: *"I trained the same as Dorian Yates, but what was good for Dorian was not as good for me. I need more sets, more volume. I grow best with 12 to 15 sets per bodypart."* – Jean-Pierre Fux

Learn from others initially: *"You will find that your greatest muscle gains will be made at the start of your training. But you must be guided through your early workouts to avoid injuries and keep muscle strains to a minimum. Training by trial and error is definitely out."* – Lou Ferrigno

Develop your mind as you develop your physique: *"You'll steadily build and strengthen your mental foundation so the ideals that instinctively drive the champions are available to you on demand."* – Peter Siegel

Routines do not always have to be the same: *"Sometimes I train just one body-part per workout and sometimes two to four different muscles per workout."* –Victor Richards

Moving to the maximum once you have warmed up: *"After I've done 2 or 3 warm-up sets, I'll go right up to my heaviest set. Keeping the reps in the 6 to 10 range for the upper body works well. For lower body I'll do anywhere from 8 to 20 reps. My lower body responds excellently to higher reps."* – Dorian Yates

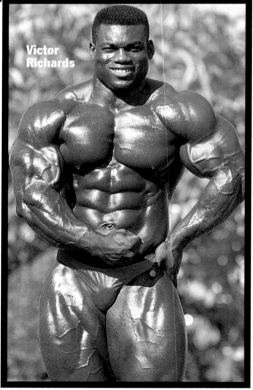

Victor Richards

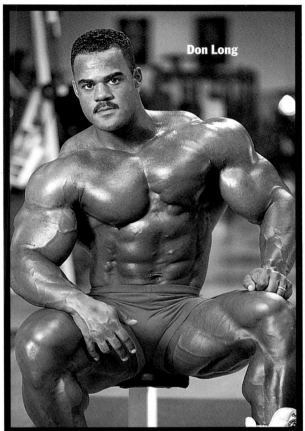

Don Long

On always learning: *"Even though I'm a professional bodybuilder, I'm still learning. You have to keep an open mind or you'll never improve."* – Jay Cutler

On workout partners: *"There's never been a time when I haven't worked with at least one partner. I currently train with three different guys ... they support and motivate me in my workouts."* – Don Long

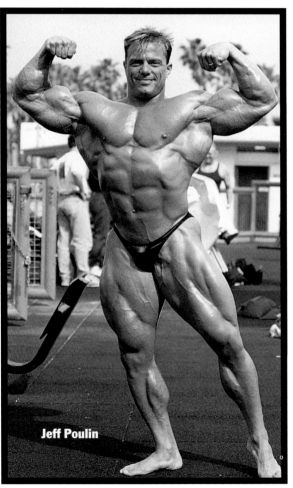

Jeff Poulin

More on training partners: *"My schedule is the main reason I don't train with a partner. Also, when I train I don't like interruptions. Whenever I've had a training partner it's been okay at first, but then he gets comfortable and wants to talk about the day's events. The conversation just gets to be distracting. A major reason why I don't train with a partner is, I train instinctively. I like to train when I have the energy. If I have to wait around until 6:00 at night for someone to get off work, that just slows me down."* – Jeff Poulin

And more: *"I like to work by myself because I can go at my own pace on days when I need to."* – Jay Cutler

3
EATING TO PRODUCE
MUSCLE GROWTH

Food has a major impact upon the human physique. The condition of the body is influenced by two primary factors – diet and exercise. When resolving to get in shape, the general public has a tendency to focus on diet, often to the exclusion of exercise. On the other hand, many novice trainers get excited about lifting iron and tend to focus totally on the exercise aspect with no concern for diet. Veterans in the sport of bodybuilding, however, have made their best gains by addressing both elements in their training program simultaneously. This chapter is dedicated to the crucial element of diet, and more specifically the nutritional approach necessary to build muscle. A diet can help or hinder the musclebuilding process. Therefore you must learn how to eat to produce muscle growth. You can't just gobble down a little more meat or cut calories to a certain level and expect to succeed. Instead, a sound nutritional approach that will enhance the muscle growth process must include well-planned strategy and a more comprehensive program.

There is strong debate over which aspect of musclebuilding is

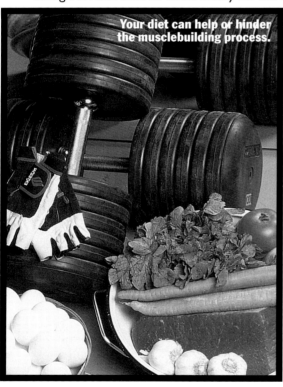

Your diet can help or hinder the musclebuilding process.

"Good training and good food come first. Those two alone are the foundation on which everything else in bodybuilding is built."
– Ronnie Coleman

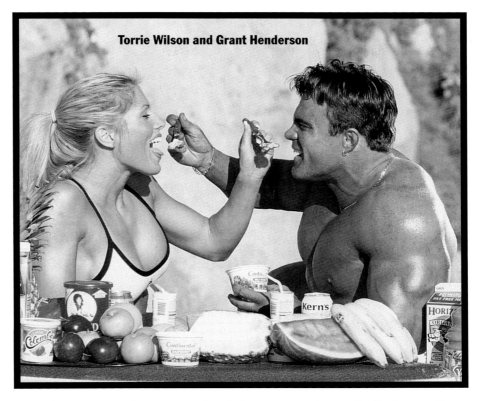

Torrie Wilson and Grant Henderson

more important – diet or exercise. It is a moot point, really. Both contribute roughly equally to the condition of the muscles and the display of those muscles on the physique. Multi-Mr. Olympia Ronnie Coleman notes: "Good training and good food come first. Those two alone are the foundation on which everything else in bodybuilding is built."

"Muscle definition doesn't occur if your bodyfat is higher than 8 to 10 percent."
– Dr. Dan Gwartney

Writer for *Ironman* bodybuilding magazine Daniel Gwartney, MD was asked what exercises are necessary to bring about a split in the biceps muscle. His answer provides real insight on the importance of both exercise and diet. "Exercising discipline in your diet is the only way you'll ever see a split in your biceps. Muscle definition doesn't occur if your bodyfat is higher than 8 to 10 percent."

How true that is, and how important the combination of diet and exercise. The exercise stimulates the muscle to grow; a good diet fuels that growth, and strips off the fat that covers the muscle. Everyone has muscle – it's just that most people's muscles are underdeveloped and obscured by bodyfat. Diet plays a big role in both developing the muscle and preventing fat from accumulating over the muscles.

Food Intake: Positive or Negative?

Food intake itself is neutral and something that everyone must do every day to survive. The food we eat can be used in a positive or negative manner. Diet is a two-edge sword that can cut in one of two ways. Diet can harm the body by allowing the accumulation of bodyfat with the related diseases that follow (heart disease, diabetes, and a host of other illnesses), or diet can fuel the hard workouts, rebuild the muscles, strip off bodyfat, as well as benefit the overall health of the body.

"Nutrition is #1 in determining how your body feels and looks."
– Laurie Vaniman

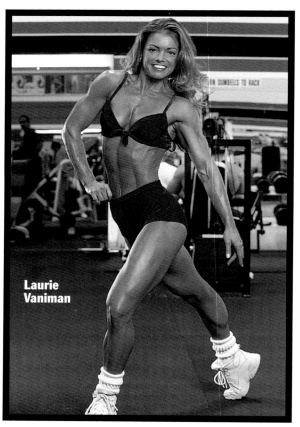

Laurie
Vaniman

Multiple Approaches

There are many ways to structure your dietary intake in order to change the shape of your physique and fuel muscle growth. As with training systems, not everyone agrees and certain routines work better for some people than for others. Additionally, there are different types of diets, depending upon the goal. The main dietary approach, is to burn off bodyfat (to an extreme degree when one is preparing for a competition). Another dietary aim, frequently in the off-season, is to add a lot more muscle mass. Each of these two goals requires a different dietary approach. Finally, there is the central concept of simultaneously building muscle and losing bodyfat — the two channels in the bodybuilding river.

Before getting started on checking out the meal arrangements and food-selection choices of the top bodybuilders, there is one stipulation: You must check with your physician first about dietary choices listed in this book if you have a known physical problem such as low or high blood sugar, heart disease, or other complications.

Build Muscle & Lose Fat?

Is that possible? Can you build muscle and lose fat at the same time? Bodybuilding star Skip La Cour says *yes*. As he points out, for building muscle, heavy training with a focus on consistent overload is required. At the same time fat can be burned off via the diet. He notes that a diet should be high in quality protein but low in fat. However, he points to "carbohydrate control" as the key to fat-burning. Skip manipulates his diet by eating only vegetables for carbs for a few days. Then he switches over to grains such as rice, pasta, and starchy veggies like potatoes for a couple of days. After that he rotates back to the veggies and protein. He has found this approach to be very effective in the pursuit of fat loss while building muscle.

"The best way to lose bodyfat is to restrict your carbohydrates in a rotating fashion."
– Skip La Cour

Skip's approach is just one of many options. Diet strategy is as important as workout strategy. Experiment with different eating styles to find out what works best for your own body. Skip has found carbohydrate manipulation to be effective for keeping his physique lean but muscular. The ways in which some bodybuilders choose to manipulate their carbs can vary greatly. Others who simply take strict control of their fat intake have had success with that technique.

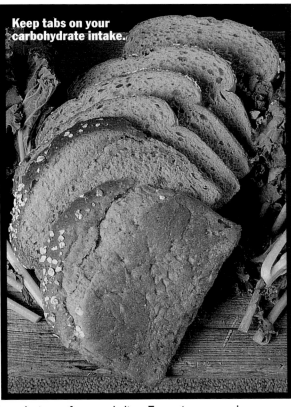

Keep tabs on your carbohydrate intake.

The following is a "cafeteria selection" of several different approaches found to be successful. Pick what you want to try and pass on the others. Some of the food combinations may shock you, particularly the intake of eggs. However, these dietary strategies have successfully turned out the hottest muscle physiques on the planet. I have featured many different meal plans as well as various foods that form the foundation of a good diet. Experiment and find what works for building your body. If one strategy is not working, try something else.

Carbohydrate manipulation is one effective manner in which to control the fat level of your physique.

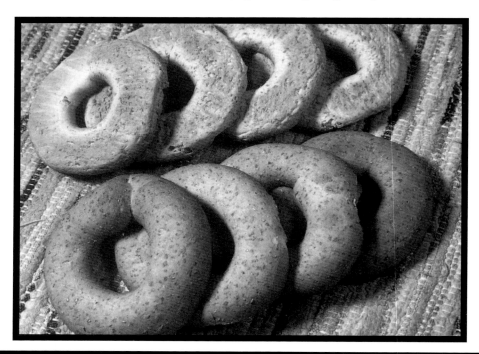

Timing and Frequency are Important

Two more elements to be aware of when perusing possible dietary strategies are the timing of dietary intake and the number of times during the day food is consumed. Why are the timing and frequency of meals important? Bodybuilding columnist Jerry Brainum points out:

"People interested in promoting an anabolic effect in muscle are often advised to eat small meals at frequent, regular intervals. The usual advice involves getting some form of protein at least every two and a half hours to maintain optimal amino acid plasma levels, which promote the positive nitrogen retention most conducive to muscular growth. In practice many bodybuilders try to eat four to eight small meals daily, which may not consist of solid foods but may instead be some type of protein drink. Eating smaller meals more often is a good idea for several reasons. Besides maintaining a more positive nitrogen balance, smaller meals also allow you to eat more calories per day with less chance of bodyfat synthesis. Studies have repeatedly shown that the identical number of calories divided over four or more meals results in less bodyfat gain than the same calories consumed in two meals. That has to do with a more controlled insulin release. Large meals promote greater insulin release, and insulin, in turn, favors storing calories as fat."

In addition to the favorable insulin effect brought about by eating more frequently (but smaller meals), another factor plays a role – the thermodynamics of eating. When you have a meal the body has to fire up its power plant to digest the food. Several processes are involved. The stomach, liver, pancreas and intestines have to produce digestive enzymes. Also involved are the storing of nutrients and elimination. This process is known to use up considerable calories. The more frequently the thermal effect of eating is cranked up, the more calories are burned off. That's another reason for having several small meals during the day instead of three larger ones – it's better for building muscle while burning off fat.

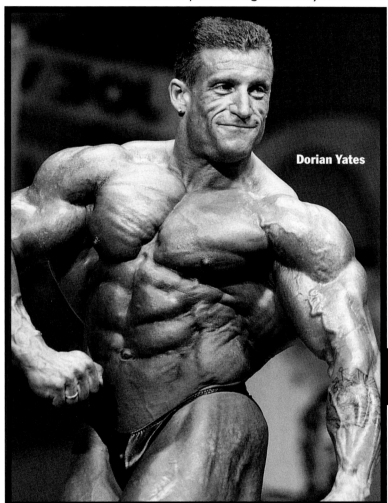

Dorian Yates

Almost all top bodybuilding professionals now enjoy the benefits of eating smaller meals frequently, timed two to three hours apart. Review the menus listed and learn to control these factors to your advantage.

Dorian Yates's Off-Season Diet

Dorian Yates spaces his meals out and eats every two to three hours. He starts the morning at around 8:00 a.m. with 7 ounces of oatmeal, 10 to 12 egg whites (with 2 or 3 yolks), a banana, a couple of pieces of whole-wheat toast, and vitamin/mineral tablets. Next comes his preworkout meal, which consists of a mixed protein/carb powder. The postworkout meal is 8 ounces of turkey, 5 ounces of rice, sweet potatoes, sweet corn, veggies and amino acid tablets. A few hours later he eats 7 ounces of tuna, 5 ounces of rice, a salad, baked potato, water and vitamin/mineral tablets. Dorian takes his fifth meal around 7:30 p.m. He gets 8 ounces of steak, baked potato, mixed veggies, water and more aminos. Around 10:00 p.m. or so he finishes the day with 7 ounces of oatmeal, 8 to 10 egg whites, water and amino acids. Note that this is his off-season diet. It lets him gain weight at a slow pace. His physique is provided with roughly 5,500 calories a day. In reviewing this daily menu, you may notice a lot of egg whites, oatmeal and meats of various sources, as well as consistent water and amino acid.

That calorie count is similar to the amount used by rising star Aaron Maddron, who tries to average about 5,500 calories a day. His aim is to take in a lot of quality protein. Aaron eats primarily animal protein, plus rice, potato, oatmeal and veggies for carbs. Breakfast includes 6 egg whites and 6 whole eggs plus a pound of red meat during the day (in lean form such as flank steak). He alternates his menu with chicken.

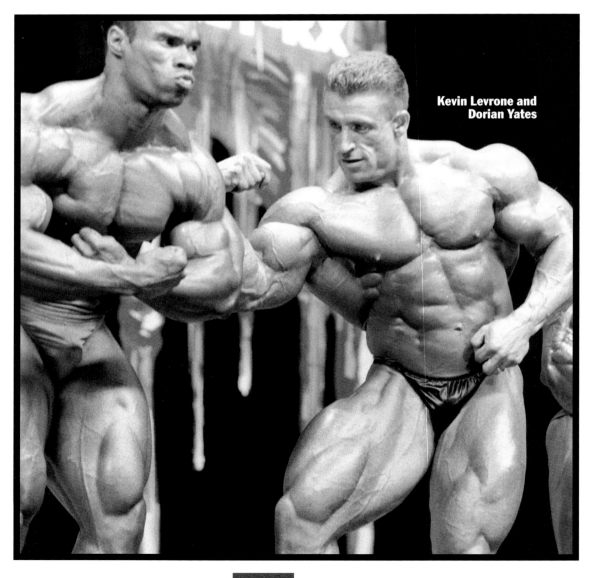

Kevin Levrone and
Dorian Yates

Natural Musclebuilding Menu

Peter Nielsen, Mr. International Universe and holder of dozens of other titles, is a natural bodybuilder who relies on a specific training diet. As he reveals in his inspirational book *Will of Iron*, Nielsen does not consume nearly as many calories as Dorian Yates, but he does space his meals out in a similar fashion over two to three hour intervals. Nielsen's diet looks like this:

Breakfast 5:00 a.m.	10 egg whites
Second breakfast 7:30 a.m.	1/3 cup oatmeal cooked in water or four rice cakes
Midmorning snack 10:30 a.m.	One broiled chicken breast and one frozen banana
Lunch 1:00 p.m.	Two chicken breasts chopped up into a salad with one cup steamed green beans, one sliced tomato, alfalfa sprouts, one tablespoon flax oil, vinegar to taste – or two whole chicken breasts with a small pasta salad
Midafternoon snack 3:00 p.m.	One protein shake including two tablespoons egg white protein powder, one cup apple juice and three ice cubes, mixed in a blender
Dinner 6:00 p.m.	One 6-ounce piece of broiled or roasted chicken or fish, 1/2 cup steamed broccoli, one baked potato or corn on the cob, spinach salad

Nielsen notes this menu works great at keeping him muscular but lean. As you can see, each meal is approximately every two to three hours. He includes both fruit and vegetables, as well as plenty of quality protein and some carbs. Notice also that he makes use of a protein shake in the afternoon with simple but effective ingredients.

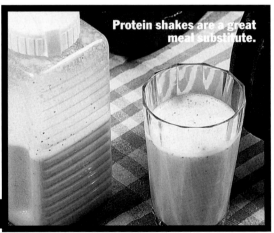

Protein shakes are a great meal substitute.

Shake It Up

Protein shakes are a great source of quality protein in a low-calorie format, and a quick way to load up on needed nutrition. If you want to incorporate a great-tasting protein shake into your diet, consider the following creation of fitness chef Jim Shiebler.

Jim Shiebler's Banana-Strawberry Cheesecake Supreme Protein Shake

2 scoops of vanilla-flavored whey protein powder
1/2 a ripe banana, peeled and sliced
2 medium strawberries, washed, stemmed and sliced
1 ounce of nonfat cream cheese
1 square of light graham cracker
1 teaspoon on honey (organic is recommended)
16 ounces of nonfat organic milk
2 or 3 cubes of ice

Put the banana, strawberries, cream cheese, honey, milk and ice cubes into a blender and pulsate for a few seconds, then switch to purée. Add protein powder and graham cracker and purée until thick and creamy.

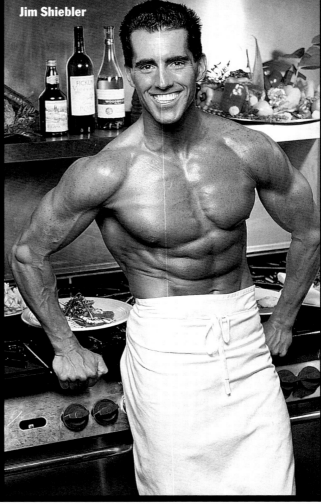

Jim Shiebler

Protein shakes are a great meal substitution as they allow for the intake of significant amounts of protein (25 to 40 grams or so) without a lot of extra fat calories or carbs. Today's high-tech protein shakes also include the full gamut of vitamins, minerals and other elements to support the body. Protein shakes can be designed in any of a thousand different ways and can be varied in calorie content with the inclusion of other blendable food items.

Bar Power

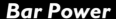

Also consider the use of protein bars. Many of those currently on the market contain 25 to 32 grams of quality protein, are low in fat, low in carbs, and contain a good amount of fiber. They taste good too. Bars come in handy for situations when you are unable to get a meal, a blender is not available, and you need nutrition. A protein bar is a tasty treat. It's a good idea to take one to the movie theater as a substitute for the empty junk calories they offer. Make sure to choose a protein bar that does not rely on white sugar as its primary source of carbohydrates.

Learn from the Ladies

Female muscle and fitness athletes do not have the great muscle size that the men do; however, the ladies seem to have a better handle on diet than most men. You can learn a ton by observing the dietary approach of female muscle athletes. Yes, if you're a guy you may need more calories during the day, but you can simply adjust by increasing the suggested serving size. The menu template a muscle lady uses can give you some excellent ideas for your own nutritional intake. Here is a good example of a great daily menu.

Heather Foster's Definition Diet

6 a.m.	6 egg whites, 1 yolk, 1 cup of oatmeal with distilled water
9 a.m.	protein shake with distilled water
12 noon	8 to 12 ounces of chicken breast (you can substitute fish, tuna or turkey), 1 cup of rice, pasta or 1 medium potato, herbal tea or distilled water
3 p.m.	protein shake with distilled water
6 p.m.	10 to 12 ounces of lean steak, salad or 1 medium potato, herbal tea or distilled water
9 p.m.	protein shake with distilled water

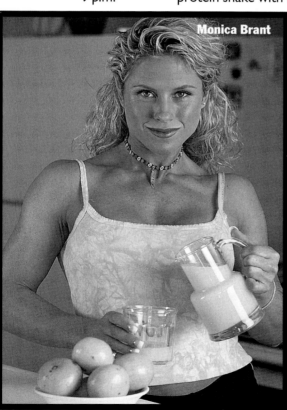

Monica Brant

Heather's diet provides plenty of protein in steady intervals, some carbs (mainly complex) and veggies as well. The low-calorie, low-fat approach is maintained in the protein drink by using water instead of milk. If you are trying to add a bit of muscle size, use milk as the base; if you are concerned with trimming and defining, use water or diluted juice.

Frequent Visitors

Some foods appear more frequently on a typical musclebuilding diet than others. Pay attention to these frequent visitors to the menu as they are the building blocks for a solid foundation. Some items that will appear on most bodybuilders weekly plans include eggs, oatmeal, chicken, tuna, protein shakes and salads. These foods have properties that mesh well with the goals of building a lean but muscular physique.

Chicken or the Egg?

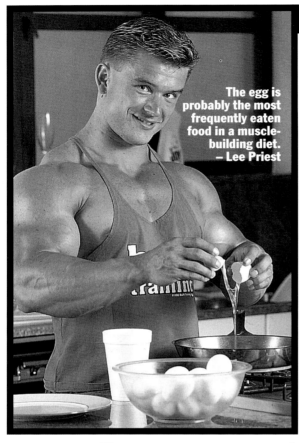

The egg is probably the most frequently eaten food in a muscle-building diet.
— Lee Priest

What came first – the chicken or the egg? For a bodybuilder both chicken and egg are highly desirable. The egg is probably the most frequently eaten food in a musclebuilding diet. And chicken, specifically chicken breast, is a close runner-up. The egg is chosen for its high protein profile. You will notice that most bodybuilders will eat only the egg white, which is almost pure protein. The egg yolk on the other hand contains fat. But don't make the mistake of throwing out all the yolks. We're talking about *good fat*. The yolk also contains protein – as much protein as the egg white. Not only that, the yolk provides vitamins and a different protein profile than the white. Together the white and yolk team up to make a powerful musclebuilding combination. The key to maximizing egg intake without pushing the fat calories too high is to eat one yolk for every two or three eggs. That way you can enjoy not only the musclebuilding benefits but also better-tasting egg meals.

The egg is a bodybuilding staple, and for good reason – the protein efficiency ratio (PER) of egg is 3.92, the highest of any food. In the PER, the higher the number the better. For example, fish has a PER of 3.55. Soy and beef both come in at 2.30. The egg is only 12 percent protein by weight (of the whole egg) but has a net *protein utilization* of 94 per-

For both chicken and turkey, choose the white meat as it has a better protein-to-fat profile.

cent, the highest of any regular food source. Fish comes in at 80 percent net protein utilization, chicken is around 70 percent, and milk measures out to 82 percent net protein utilization. Here's another factor in favor of the egg. It is much easier to eat a dozen eggs than it is to eat three or four chicken breasts. The egg is easier to eat on a continual basis and its high protein content adds up. Egg is also a good source for protein powder.

Chicken is the other half of the chicken/egg equation. Chicken, in particular chicken breast, is favored by bodybuilders since it is high in protein and low in fat, substantially lower in fat than beef and many other meats. When Dorian Yates gives his favorite sources of protein in his book *Blood and Guts*, he puts chicken at the top of the list. Peter Nielsen suggests eating a grilled chicken breast instead of a burger.

Turkey & Tuna

Turkey is closely related to chicken in that it is an excellent source of high-protein, low-fat nutrition for musclebuilding. For both chicken and turkey, choose the white meat. It has a better protein-to-fat profile. Some people miss out by eating turkey only at holidays such as Thanksgiving. Don't fall into that group. Turkey is a super food that contains great muscle-building nutrients.

Water-packed tuna is almost pure protein.

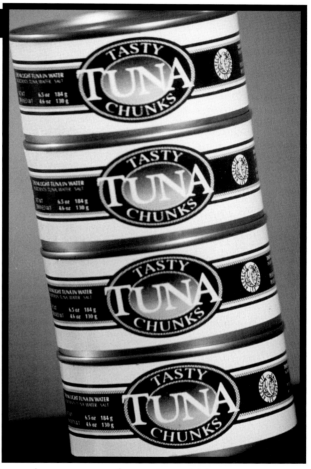

Choosing a variety of fish sources is favorable to building muscle due to the high-protein, low-fat makeup. Tuna is the most frequent choice for bodybuilders. Why tuna? Two main reasons. Tuna is cheaper than other sources of protein and it's easy to prepare. You can eat tuna right out of the can if you are in a big enough hurry. Indeed, one of the most interesting sights at past bodybuilding competitions taking place in foreign nations is one of bodybuilders lugging their cases of tuna around. Tuna is high in protein, low in fat and low in carbs. If you add it up correctly, that translates into the fact that tuna is almost pure protein. When including tuna in your diet, use the water-packed version. The oil-packed tuna is dripping in fat – not the natural fat of the fish, but a nasty partially hydrologized sort. Many find the taste of tuna to be unpleasant once ingested meal after meal. The key is to find a low-sodium, low-calorie flavor booster. Here's a suggestion.

Mix your tuna into a bowl of low-sodium instant rice and beans. Pesto and other flavorings such as low-fat/low-carb salad dressings can be used to spice up the flavor of tuna.

Tuna is not the only fish that is good for the physique. In fact most fish dishes are very good for you. Some take more time to prepare but are worth the effort both taste-wise and health-wise. Salmon is one of the very best sources of proteins and favorable omega oils for a healthy heart. Shrimp and lobster are high in protein, low in fat. You almost can't miss with fish. The following chart indicates why.

Fish (6-ounce serving)	Protein	Fat
Salmon	44 grams	14 grams*
Shrimp	44 grams	4 grams
Blue crab	38 grams	2 grams
Cod	38 grams	2 grams
Flounder	40 grams	2 grams
Haddock	40 grams	2 grams
Halibut	44 grams	4 grams
Lobster	40 grams	2 grams
Pollock	42 grams	2 grams
Rainbow trout	44 grams	8 grams
Tuna in water	36 grams	3 grams
Scallops	58 grams	2 grams
Tuna in oil	36 grams	36 grams
Sole	42 grams	2 grams

*The fat in tuna is beneficial to the heart (omega oils)

Did you know that the average seafood choice contains only 9% total calories from fat, which is even lower than both light turkey (12%) and chicken breast (20%)?

Look at the amount of protein shrimp and scallops pack – scallops at an incredible 58 grams per 6-ounce serving, and shrimp at 44 grams per 6-ounce serving. Many types of fish have only 2 grams of fat per 6-ounce serving, or 1 gram per 3-ounce serving. Who says you're stuck with tuna if you want to use fish as part of your diet? A number of different fish provide some of the best food options available to the bodybuilder. These choices have an extremely high protein/fat ratio and the fat you do get from the fish is good for your body. The average serving of seafood contains only 9 percent total calories from fat, even lower than light turkey (12 percent) and chicken breast (20 percent). In fact they average approximately 21 grams of protein for every gram of fat. This 21-to-1 ratio of protein to fat is hard for any other food to beat. The carbohydrate content in fish is almost nonexistent as well.

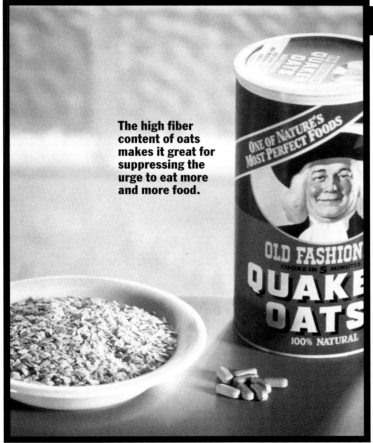

The high fiber content of oats makes it great for suppressing the urge to eat more and more food.

Oatmeal

Oatmeal is a great food to put into frequent rotation in a diet. Oats are a good source of complex carbohydrates and fiber, and are high in protein for a cereal. Conversely, oatmeal is low in fat and nil in sugars. The high fiber content of oats makes it great for suppressing the urge to eat more and more food. Oatmeal can taste bland so a very light touch of honey or molasses (which is high in B vitamins and minerals) can make it go down easier. Oatmeal is a wonder food that actually keeps your body healthy. The US Food and Drug Administration (FDA) recently released the first ever food-specific health claim, noting that, "Soluble fiber from oats as a part of a diet low in saturated fat and cholesterol may reduce the risk of heart disease." Johns Hopkins Medical Institute research found that people who regularly eat one small bowl of oatmeal have lower blood pressure than those who eat less. They found that the higher the intake of oats, the lower the blood pressure. That is just one of the variety of wonderful benefits that oats provide.

The American Cancer Society promotes eating oats as it lowers LDL (bad cholesterol) levels without lowering HDL (good cholesterol) levels. The soluble fiber, particularly in oats and barley, slows starch digestion, which may help diabetics avoid steep rises in blood sugar levels following meals. Oats are rich in B vitamins, which act as a nerve tonic and antidepressant. Oats slow the digestion of starch and are high in fiber – a great choice for the bodybuilder who wants to put the brakes on the body's insulin release.

Top Banana

The banana is a fruit that some bodybuilders use in their diet. One past veteran of the sport built up impressive size merely by greatly increasing his dietary intake of bananas. He ate large amounts every day on top of his regular intake. The banana contains fiber, vitamins, minerals, and even a little protein. Its strong suit is the potassium that it richly provides, which the body desperately needs after a workout.

Sweet & Plain Potatoes

Another great source of potassium is the potato. The potato really has no fat (unless you doctor it up with sour cream and such), has some protein, and tastes good with a meat dish. The potato is composed primarily of complex carbohydrates.

The potato's cousin, the sweet potato is a food that bodybuilders have taken to like a duck to water. The sweet potato provides a gram of fiber, two grams of protein, and various minerals and vitamins. The sweet potato does not deliver quite as much potassium as the potato, but has a lot more vitamin A. Bodybuilders are fond of the sweet potato as a prime source of complex carbohydrates that give the body a slow burn for sustained energy.

The potato is composed primarily of complex carbohydrates.

Salads & Veggies

The body needs a consistent intake of salads and vegetables to provide the full range of vitamins, minerals and roughage necessary to function at 100 percent. The recommended amount of vegetables (and fruits) is at least five servings a day. You should get at least that much no matter what type of diet you are on. And if your body is not healthy it cannot maximize your muscle mass.

Food Hall of Fame

These foods are frequent visitors to a bodybuilder's diet, and should become the foundation of your own weekly intake. Other foods to also include in the diet are nonfat yogurt, corn, beans, carrots, rice, spinach, broccoli, cauliflower, celery, apples, grapefruit, olives, barley, cabbage, low-fat or nonfat cottage

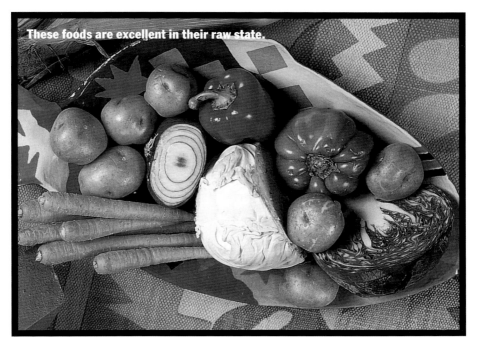

These foods are excellent in their raw state.

cheese, figs, kiwi fruit, melons, lettuce (various types), onions, mushrooms, tomatoes, nuts, pumpkin seeds, sunflower seeds, blackberries and strawberries. Add to that the cereals shredded wheat, cream of wheat and Zoom. These various items give the diet more room for change. Note that these foods are excellent in their raw state.

One of the best ways to make your meals more enjoyable is to learn how to make foods taste better without adding fats.

The general public tends to saturate some veggies in fats or thick cheese sauces. They also tend to pour sugar over cereal and high-calorie/high-fat dressing over salads and veggies. Take care in preparing your food. The bodybuilder's preparation of meats such as chicken includes removal of the skin, and grilling or broiling instead of frying. Bake your potatoes, for example, and skip the butter and sour cream. One of the best ways to make your meals more enjoyable is to learn how to make foods taste better without adding fats. The use of certain types of nonfat and low-sodium spices and other flavor enhancements (molasses on cereals, for example) goes a long way toward sustaining a dietary approach. Nonfat, low-carb dressings are another dietary tool that can be used to enhance the flavor of foods. If you do use oils, use canola oil and olive oil. A diet that always consists of the same few elements not only lacks full nutrient coverage, but also can become quite boring. A diet should be tight, but it doesn't have to be boring.

Are you still stumped on putting together a new daily menu? Here are a few more ideas to spark your imagination.

Joe Spinello's Super Diet

Breakfast 7 a.m.	10 scrambled egg whites, 1 cup of oatmeal and water, multivitamins and supplements
Before workout	supplements
Morning snack	(1/2 hour after training) 2 scoops of MVP Labs Pro Whey with water, 10 grams of MVP Glutamate
Lunch 12 noon	8 ounces of broiled chicken breast, 8 ounces of baked potato, 2 cups of steamed veggies, supplements
Snack 3 p.m.	2 scoops of Pro Whey in water (preferably chocolate)
Dinner 6 p.m.	8 ounces of baked or grilled chicken, 8 ounces baked potato, 2 cups of steamed veggies, multivitamins and supplements
Evening snack 9 p.m.	12 egg white omelet, supplements

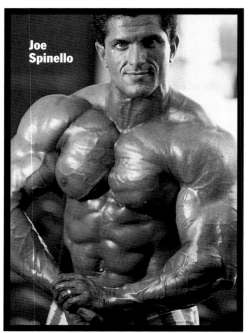

Joe Spinello

Even though his diet is narrowly built around chicken, baked potatoes and egg whites, Joe still gets in several servings of vegetables every day.

Lou's Incredible Weight Gainer

Big Lou Ferrigno, the Incredible Hulk, recommends the following diet in his latest book, *Guide to Personal Power*:

Meal one 8 a.m.	Cheese omelet with 4 or 5 eggs, whole-grain toast, 1 piece of fruit, 1 or 2 glasses of whole milk
Meal two 11 a.m.	2 meat or cheese sandwiches on whole-grain bread, 3 ounces of raw nuts, 1 or 2 glasses of whole milk
Meal three 2 p.m.	Tuna salad, piece of fresh fruit sliced over yogurt, 1 or 2 glasses of whole milk
Meal four 5 p.m.	1 protein drink consisting of 1 pint of whole milk, 1/3 cup of milk and egg protein powder and fruit or another flavoring for taste
Meal five 8 p.m.	Steak, vegetable, baked potato, 1 or 2 glasses of whole milk
Meal six 11 p.m.	3 ounces of hard cheese, 3 ounces of raw sunflower seeds, 1 or 2 glasses of whole milk (as an alternative, another protein drink)

Not only does Lou's suggested size-gaining diet supply a lot of protein and calories, it is also well rounded with fruit, veggies, nuts and dairy products. Many of the food choices he lists are specific to weight gaining only and are not applicable to a trimming diet. His suggested diet for cutting bodyfat is quite different:

Meal one 8 a.m.	10 egg whites, medium bowl of oatmeal with a handful of raisins, 8 to 12 ounces of water, 1 multivitamin/mineral tablet
Meal two 11:15 a.m.	1 chicken breast, big bowl of brown rice, fruit platter (mainly melons and bananas), half a tuna sandwich on whole-wheat bread
Meal three 2:30 p.m.	2 chicken breasts, medium-size bowl of brown and white rice mixed
Meal four 5 p.m.	1 chicken breast mixed in with 6 egg whites, cooked with a nonfat spray served on a bed of rice, 1 multivitamin/mineral supplement, 1 glass of water
Meal five 8:30 p.m.	6 to 8 ounce turkey breast cut into strips and mixed in with 6 egg whites, onions and bell peppers, large helping of mixed vegetables, water

Notice Lou included some raisins in the oatmeal – not a bad idea. They supply extra vitamins, minerals and flavor to the bland oatmeal. Also notice Lou uses onions and bell peppers to add zest to his evening meal. This is a great way to make the foods tastier without additional fats or sugars.

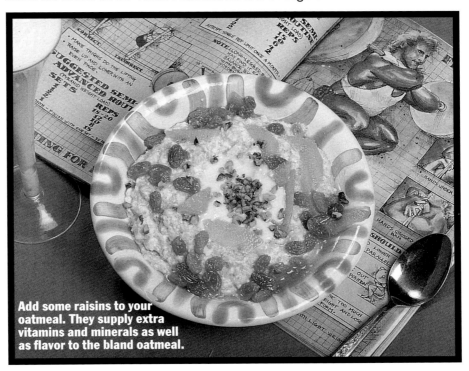

Add some raisins to your oatmeal. They supply extra vitamins and minerals as well as flavor to the bland oatmeal.

Dinner time is the wrong time to load up on water – drink it throughout the day, but not with meals.

Many bodybuilders take water with their meals. Trainer and bodybuilder Peter Nielsen points out that this is a mistake – water should be taken all day long, but not with meals. When people mention they drink tons of water with their food, Nielsen tells them that is the wrong way to consume the daily quota of water. It dilutes the food and makes for less efficient absorption of nutrients. For these reasons he advises avoiding water 15 minutes before a meal and for 30 to 60 minutes afterward. However, a large quantity of water should be taken during the rest of the day, particularly on training days.

Peter Nielsen's "Regimen for the Rail"

Consider Nielsen's menu for those who wish to gain muscle size:

Breakfast	8 egg whites, 1/2 cup of oatmeal cooked in water
Midmorning snack	(2 to 3 hours later) One 1200-calorie gainer supplement (less than one gram of fat per serving, very high in carbs)
Lunch	(2 to 3 hours later) 1/2 pound of roast beef (lean) on whole-wheat bread, green salad with tomato, 1 tablespoon oil plus vinegar (flax oil and apple cider vinegar is his choice) (good alternate lunch would be two whole 4-ounce chicken breasts and a pasta salad)
Midafternoon snack	(2 to 3 hours later) 1 protein shake: 2 tablespoons egg-white protein powder (25 grams of fat-free protein), 1 cup two percent milk, 1 tablespoon peanut butter, 1 banana and 3 ice cubes, all mixed in blender
Dinner	(2 to 3 hours later) Two 5-ounce pieces of broiled or roasted chicken or fish (whitefish, swordfish or tuna) or one 10-ounce steak, 1/2 cup steamed broccoli, 1 baked potato or corn on the cob, spinach salad

Even though the calories are higher and more protein is made available than with his main diet, this version still steers away from fat intake.

Some bodybuilders get quite extreme in their approach to diet. Monstrous Greg Kovacs, for instance, is known to be an eating machine. He aims for 16 meals a day for a daily caloric intake that tops 10,000. Lots of chicken

"Never be afraid to drink water, especially during your workouts." – Sherry Goggin-Giardina

and supplements – that's what enables him to reach the high-calorie, high-protein intake that builds his massive muscles. Most nutritionists point to the fact that the body can effectively digest only so many grams of protein per meal. One determining factor, of course, is body size. A bigger person like Kovacs can afford to take in more grams per meal than someone with a smaller body.

Here is another super protein shake idea from chef Jim Shiebler, featured in *Physical Magazine,* which provides a very hefty dose of protein:

Cran-Grape Multivitamin Blast Shake
1 package of vanilla meal-replacement powder
1 tablespoon multivitamin/mineral powder
1 ounce of frozen cranberries (approximately 8)
2 ounces of ripe seedless red grapes (about 8), washed and stemmed
1 cup of orange juice
1 cup of distilled cold water
2 ice cubes
Put the orange juice, water, ice, cranberries and grapes into the blender. Pulsate to begin with, then switch to purée. Remove the lid and carefully add meal-replacement powder and multi- vitamin/mineral powder. Purée until silky smooth. Pour into a chilled glass and enjoy. Yields one 22-ounce shake.
Nutritional value: protein 44 grams, calories 431, carbs 55, fat 5 grams.

Why the Focus on Protein?

What's all the fuss about always trying to get lots of protein? Why is there such emphasis on protein in a bodybuilding diet? Well, the key nutritional element for building the muscles is protein. Other nutrients support growth, but protein lies at the center of the process. Human muscles are mainly water, but merely taking in a lot of water won't do anything

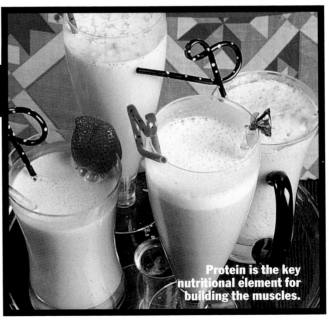

Protein is the key nutritional element for building the muscles.

Chemical composition of muscle fiber:
water = 75%
proteins = 20%
fat = 2%
salts = 2%
nitrogenous extractive and carbs = 1%
Total = 100%

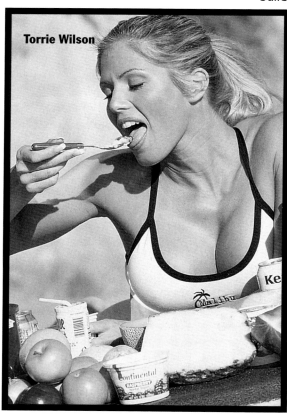

Torrie Wilson

without plenty of protein. *Gray's Anatomy* states, in chemical composition the muscular fibers may be said to consist of (in round numbers) 75 percent water, 20 percent proteins, 2 percent fat, 1 percent nitrogenous extractive and carbohydrates, and 2 percent salts, which are mainly potassium phosphate and carbonate. Of the nonwater substance in the muscles, protein is the most plentiful, and the most vital. Protein makes up roughly 74 percent of the dry weight of most body cells. A lack of adequate protein can cause the body to fall apart – literally.

The average person in a developed nation generally gets enough protein for the sedentary lifestyle most enjoy. However, the drastic process of building muscle requires more than the amount recommended for a sedentary person. Studies by Peter Lemon, PhD, indicate that athletes do indeed need more protein than sedentary individuals. Of all sports, the musclebuilding pursuit requires the most protein due to the very nature of the endeavor. Musclebuilding is a dynamic process in which the body is in a state much like that of an infant – a growth state. To facilitate the growth of muscle tissue strong protein intake is vital. Lemon found that those engaging in endurance exercise should consume 1.2 to 1.4 grams of protein per kilogram of bodyweight every day, which translates to 150 to 175 percent of the RDA. That is just for endurance athletes. The recommendation for resistance-training athletes is even higher – 1.7 to 1.8 kilograms of protein per kilogram of bodyweight. That translates to 212 to 225 percent of the present RDA. Bodybuilders have known they need more protein than the average Joe for years. Most will use a rule of thumb of 1 to 1.5 grams of protein for every pound of bodyweight. In fact that is what Ronnie Coleman lists on his Web site: "Consume 1.5 grams of protein per pound of bodyweight per day." Bodybuilders are unique in their protein needs.

> ## *"I never had a problem with eating because I didn't keep sweets in the house." – Cory Everson*

Athletes in other sports are not necessarily trying to build up the size of their muscles. They are trying to do some action (like put a ball in a hoop, a puck in a net, etc.). Therefore they do not need the high flow of protein a bodybuilder does.

Protein should come from quality sources (one that supplies all the essential amino acids) on a consistent basis. Protein can also be used as a source of energy, but you want to avoid this state as much as possible, letting fats and carbs serve as fuel sources. A carbohydrate diet that is too low can lead to the necessity of proteins being broken down and used as a fuel source, a catabolic condition.

Remember, the best sources of protein are eggs, fish, whey, poultry (chicken, turkey, etc.), meat and dairy products. Protein often comes grouped

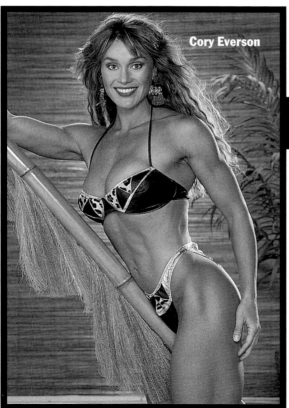

Cory Everson

with fats and it is a good idea to separate the two before having the protein. Choose nonfat cottage cheese or lean cuts of beef such as flank steak.

Carbs – High or Low Levels?

The main fuel source for a challenging workout is carbohydrates. Carbohydrates are converted into glycogen and this fuels the stop-and-go action of weightlifting. Carbohydrates come in several different forms that can facilitate different purposes in a training program. Complex carbohydrates are the type that burn off slowly. This is the best type of carb for fueling the body throughout the day. Complex carbs help keep insulin levels consistent. So do fibrous carbs. There are two

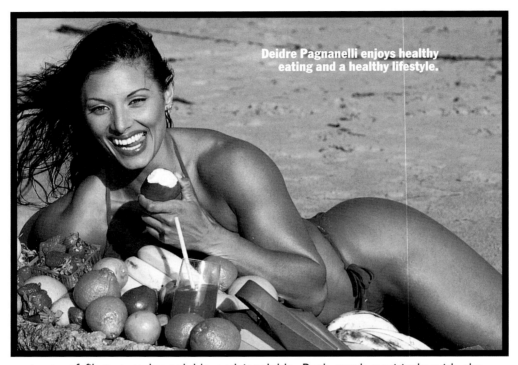

Deidre Pagnanelli enjoys healthy eating and a healthy lifestyle.

types of fibrous carbs: soluble and insoluble. Both work positively with the digestive system; conversely, a lack of fiber can cause problems and even lead to internal disease. Generally 15 to 25 grams of fiber intake a day is needed for a healthy, functioning digestive system, but in the developed nations many people who rely so much on refined foods come up short. Fiber intake improves cholesterol levels and also reduces the chance of having a heart attack. Fiber is believed to absorb fat and cholesterol from the intestines. Fiber plays an important role in the bodybuilder's diet as it satiates hunger pangs. Adding a little more fiber to the diet will take away the constant urge to eat and help guard against snacking on empty calories. Good sources of fiber include various fruits and vegetables, oats, certain cereals, rice, legumes, celery, carrots, bran and wheat germ.

The final type of carbohydrate is the simple carb, or sugar carb. Each of these carbohydrates plays a vital role in the functioning of the body. Unfortunately the average person tends to overindulge in sugar carbs. Refined flour and sugar intake (the essential ingredients in junk food) is at an all-time high, and not coincidentally so are physical ailments. What role do sugar carbs play in a bodybuilder's diet? Sugars do have a key role, but not throughout the day. Instead they have a specific positive purpose. Right after a workout is the best time to take in simple carbs. Resistance training depletes the muscle fibers of glycogen. The first type of carb to burn out is the fast-acting ATP. Then the mainstream glycogen is used up. Lack of adequate muscle glycogen can hinder training efforts: Muscle glycogen is an important energy substate during resistance-training activity, and conversely, reduced muscle glycogen impairs strength performance. Low muscle glycogen appears to accentuate exercise-induced muscle weakness.

It's a smart idea to replenish this supply right after your workout. In fact you can even start to reload the carbs during the workout. Honey has been shown to enhance the performance by repacking carb stores, as have carbohydrate-electrolyte beverages, leading to training benefits such as prolonged workouts at a higher level of intensity. Additionally, the best postworkout refueling comes from a mix of carbs and protein. Reloading the carb stores directly after your workout will affect the next workout (as will a lack of refueling in a negative manner).

Successful resistance training on a regular basis requires consistent carb refueling. There exists what has been described as a window of opportunity that is open right after a resistance workout. This window is the time frame immediately after a workout when the body more readily utilizes and stores the incoming carbs. Research has shown that by eating carbohydrates shortly after a weight-training routine the body repacks the energy lost in the workout and thus helps prepare the body for the next routine.

Generally 15 to 25 grams of fiber intake a day is needed for a healthy, functioning digestive system.

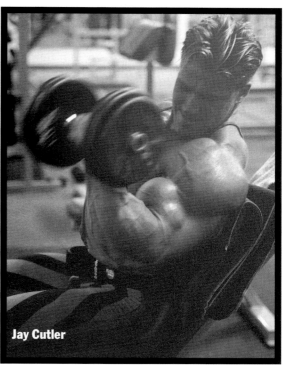

Jay Cutler

Multi-Mr. Olympia Lee Haney notes this strategy, pointing out, "Eat for what you are about to do, not for what you have done." Preparation for the next workout starts the minute the current workout ceases. The time frame specified most frequently by research as the best time to replenish carbs is 15 minutes to two hours after the workout. A researcher at the University of Toronto, Canada, has shown that a recommended dose of carbohydrates (0.5 grams of carbohydrate per pound of bodyweight) taken immediately after a workout, and again one hour after exercising has a beneficial effect on protein metabolism by way of decreasing breakdown and enhancing retention. This effect is totally beneficial for the bodybuilder. This factor has become so

Adding a little more fiber to your diet helps take away the constant urge to eat and helps guard against the urge to snack on empty calories.

acclaimed in the physique world that several supplement companies are very aware of this replenishment aspect and have come out with specific drinks and bars for refueling. These training supplements dedicated to the postworkout recovery have continued to improve as they have evolved.

Additional discoveries related to postworkout carb intake revealed that even the type of carbohydrate taken after exercise can make a difference — carbohydrates that rate high on the glycemic index (graham crackers, bread, rice cakes, carrot juice, potatoes, etc.) provide a more readily (quickly) assimilated glycogen source than do carbohydrates with a low glycemic-index rating.

Resistance training (weightlifting in particular) causes a significant decrease in muscle glycogen due to the stressful nature of the exercise. (For instance, 3 sets of biceps curls done to failure can stimulate a 25 percent reduction in muscle glycogen.) To overcome this problem, the key is to focus on replacing the lost energy stores. Failure to adequately replace this lost muscle glycogen can cause the next workout to fall short of maximal output.

Jean Storlie, MS, RD, states, "Bodies have a lot of work to do to repair

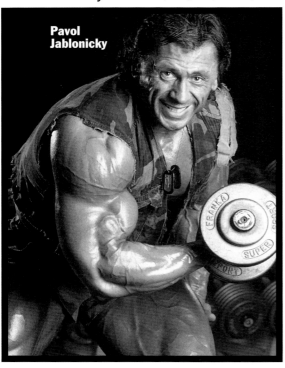

Pavol Jablonicky

tissues that took a beating during exercise and replenish depleted energy stores. In addition, during periods of intense training and competition, when there is little time to recover between workouts, post-exercise nutrition becomes an even more important factor in enhancing performance and preventing injury." Resistance training taxes the physique heavily. The nutritional elements must replace what was burned off during the workout. They must also provide for a little extra to facilitate new growth — if that is to occur. Merely replacing what was lost is not enough for musclebuilding — a little extra must be incorporated for muscle growth beyond the break-even point.

Musclebuilding concerns not only the performance of the exercises to

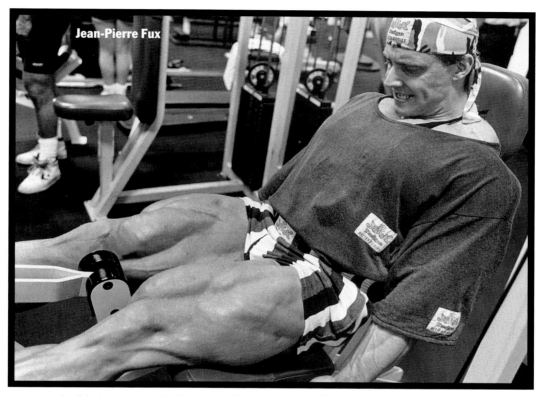

Jean-Pierre Fux

build the muscle (which is similar to almost all other athletic pursuits) but also blasting the body to a new level of muscular development in itself (which is not similar to other athletic pursuits). The emphasis on growth is somewhat exclusive to bodybuilding and must be factored into the nutrition equation as it involves more than just replenishment – it also calls for going beyond the "re" level and allowing for growth in the muscles. Refueling is most essential for the task of musclebuilding, where the intense workout thrives on a full tank, and where recovery must exceed 100 percent to include the growth factor.

The focus on replacing the muscle glycogen stores is of crucial importance for the bodybuilder if substantial muscle gains are to be made. The process of recovery can be taken a step further by adding in protein to the refueling mix.

The nutritional elements must replace what was burned off during the workout. They must also provide for a little extra to facilitate new muscle growth – if that is to occur.

Protein is not often viewed from the angle of replenishment. As noted previously, a strong intake of protein is needed for muscle growth. Eating protein throughout the day is necessary for muscle growth. However, taking protein after a taxing workout is also very important. Studies have shown that the availability of free amino acids immediately following exercise increased muscle anabolism by increasing protein synthesis and decreasing protein breakdown. Protein is a vital recovery factor, and if you ignore it you miss out on the full potential your workout can yield. Protein intake appears to be particularly important in exercises which result in muscle damage, such as repetitive power workouts to exhaustion and eccentric movements (which produce force during muscle lengthening).

Protein repacking may be almost as vital as carb repacking. Simply replacing the carbohydrates is not enough and can cause you to miss out on full muscle recovery. Research shows that combining protein with carbohydrate in the post-exercise meal increases glycogen synthesis. University of Illinois nutrition professor Donald Layman points out that taking the amino acid leucine right after training can shorten the down time your body needs between workouts.

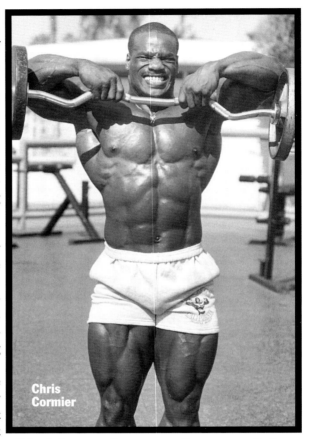

Chris Cormier

Taking the amino acid leucine right after training can shorten the down time your body needs between workouts.

Studies reveal that when leucine was ingested within 15 minutes of the completion of the last set of a workout, the leucine appeared to quick-start the protein rebuilding process – indicating that muscles can recover more quickly, and the body can be better prepared for the next round of heavy exercise. Leucine is one of the essential amino acids, meaning it cannot be synthesized by the body but must always be acquired from dietary sources. The good news about leucine is that it is present in all protein foods. It is available in strong concentrations in meat and dairy products, and to a minor degree in wheat germ, brown rice, soybeans, almonds,

The best time to repack your muscle glycogen is during the "window of opportunity" which occurs from 15 minutes to two hours after your workout.

cashews, brazil nuts, corn, lentils and chickpeas. Leucine is fantastic because it inhibits the breakdown of muscle proteins. Leucine also stimulates protein synthesis in muscles, and is essential for growth, promoting the healing of bones, skin and muscle tissue. Bodybuilders should be informed that leucine promotes postworkout muscle recovery.

You must obtain carbs and some protein within the time period directly after a workout – particularly during the 15 minute to two-hour "window of opportunity." The type of carbs taken at this point should have a specific glycemic makeup.

Glycemic Index

One of the most important factors of consideration in the carbs/training mix is the glycemic index. The glycemic index is a measurement tool used to determine how fast blood sugar reacts to certain types of foods. *Avery's Sports Nutrition Almanac* points out that the index indicates the metabolic consequences of ingestion of different types of foods. The *Almanac* notes: "It is better to consume foods with a low glycemic index for meals and snacks, since these help maintain the proper blood sugar level and ensure a sustained energy supply. Conversely, during workouts and competitions it is better to eat foods with a high glycemic index because they will help spare glycogen in the body and supply quick energy to exercising muscles."

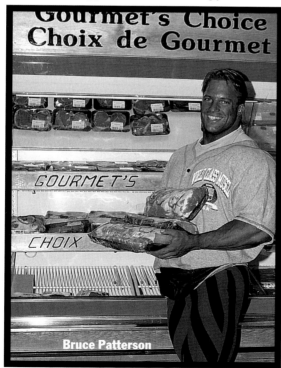

Bruce Patterson

Most of the time you want to eat low glycemic index carbs such as apples, beans and soybeans. Surprisingly, milk and milk products have a low glycemic index rating and are better for sustained energy release. (Yes, ice cream is a slow inducer of insulin secretion! For slow insulin release, ice cream is much better than whipped potatoes, for example.) Mix in some fiber and complex carbs and you can get the slow release of energy that works best during the day. But for a workout you want energy from the carbs available right away. The best foods for this are carrots, cornflakes, honey, potatoes, breads, maltose and rice. Glucose itself has the highest glycemic-index rating. To facilitate the quick energy release, consider the glycemic blast after a workout.

Fat puts the brakes on rapid induction of insulin secretion so avoid mixing fat with high glycemic index sources for the initial postworkout recovery.

Glycemic Blast

Most stores sell carrot juice. Some top physique stars from the past such as Steve Reeves drank carrot juice for health benefits. Carrot juice is near the very top of the glycemic index and makes a great postworkout drink. Add to the

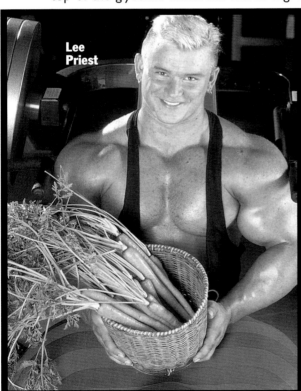

Lee Priest

effect with other high glycemic index food items like graham crackers and honey. This unique combination taken after a workout will repack your glycogen very quickly. Put the honey on the graham crackers and drink the carrot juice for a real jolt. But I warn you — buy the low-fat or nonfat graham crackers, if possible, to skirt the slowdown as fat puts the brakes on rapid induction of insulin secretion.

How Many Grams?

How many carbs should you take after a workout? Most research points to getting at least 75 grams of carbs to fully replace those lost over the course of a workout lasting more than half an hour.

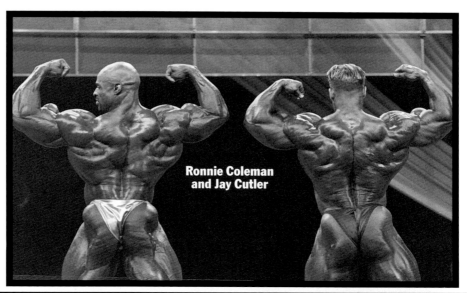

Ronnie Coleman
and Jay Cutler

Low Carb Cycle

A low carb cycle can provide an effective short-term manner in which to burn off bodyfat. When the carbs are low, the body turns to fat as a fuel source and carves off those extra pounds you have hanging around. However, don't drop the carb intake too low. (Lee Haney notes 30 percent of total caloric value as the lower range.) Lowering the carbs too low and/or going on a low-carb diet for too long can cause your body to start burning *precious muscle* as a fuel source – a disaster you definitely don't want to see happen. If you use a low-carb diet, strictly monitor your muscles (with tape measure on biceps, chest and thighs) to ensure the weight loss is coming from the fat. Don't overdo the low-carb diet approach – use it for a short cycle in certain phases, then back off.

All fats have a high calorie-per-gram count.

Carbohydrates are vital for the right flow of energy – slow and sustained release during the day; fast action during and after a workout. Manipulate your carbohydrate intake to control your energy levels to suit your training and recovery.

Fats – Friend & Foe

Dietary fat is both friend and foe in the musclebuilding process. Fat is necessary and good; too much fat is bad. Not only does too much fat intake accumulate over the muscles, it also harms the health of the body. Some fat is necessary in the diet, and some fats are essential because they are very much needed by the body.

As with carbohydrates, fats are divided into different groups. Fats are known as lipids – in the plural, as there is more than one type. Some you want in your diets; others you want to avoid. Avery's *Sports Nutrition Almanac* notes, "Certain lipids are essential to health … Rather than cut lipids out of your diet completely, you should learn how to balance the good lipids with the bad lipids in your diet and how to trim total lipid intake." The *Almanac* also notes that power athletes are more prone to becoming fat because of the differential use of energy sources – an endurance athlete such as a long distance runner does use a lot of fat as a fuel source due to the length of the training session; the power

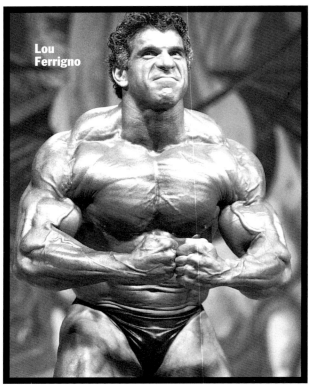

Lou Ferrigno

athlete uses carbs as the primary fuel source. This means there can be a natural tendency to accumulate too much bodyfat. Certainly not all fats are bad and the fact that Eskimos have maintained diets with an upper range of 60 percent of total caloric intake from fat without notable heart, cancer or diabetes problems is very significant. However, the fat intake equation is complex and several issues need to be weighed and balanced.

All fats (even the good ones) are dangerous in one sense due to their high calorie content. A gram of fat contains 9 calories compared to less than half that amount for carbs and protein (only 4 calories each). For this reason even good fats should not be eaten in high amounts as the calories will quickly add up. The answer is not to drop fat intake to zilch, either. Lou Ferrigno points out that, when he dropped his fat intake to almost zero he would feel weak and dizzy, and his muscles would lack fullness. He believes fats give the muscles a certain fullness. Many other trainers recommend getting a good portion of your caloric intake from fat sources – the right type of fat, of course.

Various Fats

There are a few main types of fats – triglycerides, fatty acids, cholesterol and phospholipids. Triglycerides are the major group, comprised mostly of the fats eaten and stored by the body. Of the other types, the fatty acids have familiar names – saturated fats, monounsaturated acids and polyunsaturated acids. In general it is best to avoid the saturated types. The types of fat you should try to include in your dietary intake (and supplementation if necessary) are the essential fatty acids. Linoleic acid is needed by the body for growth and general health. The omega-3 and omega-6 fatty acids are beneficial to the heart and are found most predominately in certain fish such as salmon and cod. Medium-chain triglycerides are more quickly digested and one of the fastest energy sources of the various fats. Gamma linolenic acid is another of the good fats and serves in the insulin support role, as well as helping the immune system.

How Much Fat?

How much fat should you have in your diet? There are two primary schools of thought in bodybuilding theory. One calls for an extremely low intake of fat – 10 percent or less of total calories. The other calls for a higher fat intake – anywhere from 20 to 30 percent of the total diet. Naturally if you go on a low-carbohydrate diet the difference (total caloric percentage) has to be made up somewhere and many advocate making up that difference with both protein and fats. One answer to the dilemma of the structure of a low-carb diet is to incorporate more fiber to keep the protein and fat percentages slightly lower (fiber will not be a caloric problem). You will have to experiment with fat percentage ranges to find out what works best for your body. Know that the suggested lower limit is around 10 percent, the suggested upper limit around 30 percent. Work within these guidelines and watch how your body responds. Adjust accordingly.

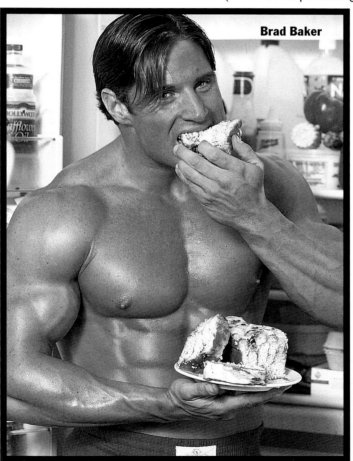

Brad Baker

Always focus any fat intake on the best sources such as flaxseed oil and fish oils. Skip the fatty cuts of meat and the heavily saturated fats in dairy products – get your fats from fish. Oils from nuts and seeds (sunflower and pumpkin seeds are especially good) are also beneficial. When cooking, use oils that are good for the body – olive oil, canola oil, etc.

Timing the Fat Intake

When you are training to build up the muscles, particularly if you're aiming at more body size and fueling the mass growth cycle (such as in off-season training), you will want to incorporate a higher percentage of fats into your diet. Fat is part of the growth process and getting rid of it entirely when trying to build up size and mass is a mistake. On the other side of the coin, for dieting down and preparing for a contest, or simply for just carving off excess weight around the waistline, move to a lower fat percentage – that's the trick. You want to limit your fat intake to 10 percent fat of your daily intake, which will drop the total calorie count. Sure, you can use a low-carb diet in a cyclical fashion to burn off fat for a specific phase, but use the low-fat diet as the main base to gravitate back to between low-carb diet cycles as you trim down.

Helpful Dietary Hints

One of the toughest aspects of building a muscular physique is adhering to a diet. The pressures of always eating in a sound nutritional manner are tough.

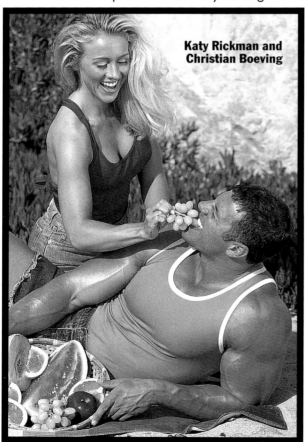

Katy Rickman and Christian Boeving

The diet is the one area where most musclebuilding programs fail. Many bodybuilders spend most of the year carrying around more than 10 percent bodyfat, obscuring the overall muscle lines and totally hiding the abdominals. If you want to be a genuine bodybuilder, you don't have to compete in a contest – instead you simply have to look the part. This means a bodyfat level of 10 percent or less, which comes from strict diet control. There is no way around it – diet is the chasm that divides the successful bodybuilder from the wannabe.

As nasty as a tight diet can be, there are some things you can do to help make it happen. The first is to recognize that, although the diet needs to be strict, it doesn't have to be so tight that you squeak. One trick many bodybuilders use is to allow themselves a junk food day on occasion.

This may be once a week, once every two weeks or once a month, depending upon the training cycle being used. The key here is to take a little pressure off your appetite. Go ahead and have a bit of chocolate or some other treat every now and then. A bowl of ice cream on the rare occasion will not prove fatal to your appearance. Keep the junk food very infrequent, but do allow yourself some treats on occasion. If you never grant your taste buds anything good they will rebel and before you know it you will be binging on all kinds of empty calories.

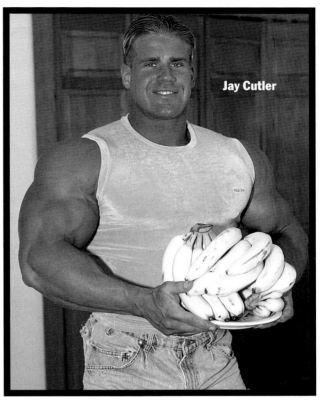

Jay Cutler

Keep the junk food very infrequent, but do allow yourself some treats on occasion.

Another helpful hint is to include some food items that are tasty but low in calories. When butter is omitted and the salt kept low, popcorn is a good treat. Nonfat salad dressings bring flavor to many foods. Molasses is another topping that adds flavor, but it is also very healthy for the body. Buy a nutrition almanac and check the food composition of everything you contemplate eating. You will find that several foods are not as bad for you as you thought. And again, spice it up to your advantage.

Diet is not everything in the musclebuilding process but without it you can lose control on everything. The body tends to accumulate fat easily while muscle gains come the hard way. Make sure your food intake gives your muscles a boost instead of being a stumbling block that will hinder your progress.

- The diet is as important as exercise for promoting muscular growth.
- Use low-carb intake in a cyclical fashion only; do not use it as a dietary base.
- Eat several small to moderate-size meals per day rather than a few big ones.
- Drink lots of water – but not at meal time.
- Aim for 25 to 40 grams of quality protein per meal.
- Do not drastically reduce fat intake if you are trying to gain size; utilize the good fats for more growth.

Thoughts From the Pros on Eating to Produce Muscle Growth

Frank Sepe

Lean & Clean: *"Every winter I take two weeks off my regular diet ritual and enjoy the holidays. Then I get back into my strict eating habits again around January 1st. During the year I cheat on Sundays. I feel that a cheat day is necessary every week to shock your system, boost your metabolism, and help you stay sane. Ever since I lost my huge muscle mass I focus more on eating clean. I stick to low calories, high protein, low carbs and low fat now, whereas I used to eat high carbs, high protein and moderate fat."*
– Frank Sepe

Out With Tradition? *"What's wrong with traditional diets? I've tried them all, and even the most medically and athletically correct diets allow much too much muscle loss. On your typical low-fat, high-carbohydrate, lose-a-pound-a-week diet you will lose one pound of muscle for every three pounds of fat! No lie!"* – the late Dan Duchaine

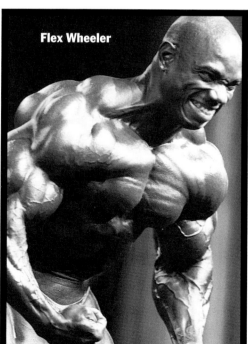

Flex Wheeler

On Taking a Break: *"I will not turn 40 having spent my life doing nothing but eating chicken and fish and grinding it out, day after day, without a break from the routine."*
– Chris Cormier

The Excellent Egg: *"When people ask me what they should eat to get big, I tell them to eat eggs."* – Chris Aceto

Dietary Application: *"You can have the best diet in the world, but if you don't follow it, it does you no good."* – Flex Wheeler

The Eating/Exercising Relationship: *"You should always space out the time you eat from the time you exercise. A good rule of thumb is not to eat at least one hour prior to the time you have scheduled to train."*
– Lou Ferrigno

Nutrient Intake: *"My carb intake during off-season is about 80 percent of my total daily caloric intake with 20 percent comprised of protein and fats. My precontest carb intake is around 80 to 250 grams per day with between 400 and 600 grams of protein per day."* – Nasser El Sonbaty

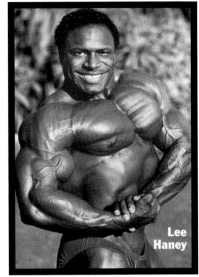

Lee Haney

On Dietary Percentages: *"Split your calories according to the following: 60 to 65 percent carbs, 15 to 30 percent proteins, 10 to 20 percent fats."* – Ronnie Coleman

Carbs for Gaining and Losing: *"Eat a diet of 60 percent carbohydrates for weight gain; about 30 percent for weight loss."* – Lee Haney

On Fats: *"We measure optimum intake (of fats) by how the skin feels. When you get the optimum amount of essential fats they form a barrier in the skin against the loss of moisture, and so they are nature's perfect moisturizer."* – Udo Erasmus, PhD, author of *Fats That Heal, Fats That Kill*

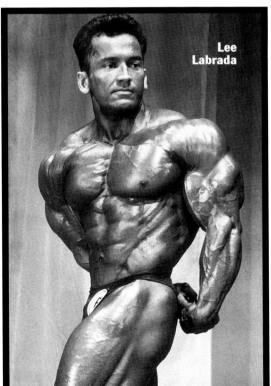

Lee Labrada

On Eating for Muscles: *"Eating six meals a day is necessary to ensure that your muscles are constantly bathed in nutrients such as amino acids."* – Lee Labrada

On Taking Responsibility: *"Are you really consuming five or six feeds daily and getting enough calories and nutrients to grow on? Are you really sleeping well for at least eight hours every night? If you can't answer yes to those questions, you have only yourself to blame for slow or nonexistent progress."* – Stuart McRobert in *Ironman* magazine

On Digestion: *"Eat plenty of greens for proper digestion."* – Mike Matarazzo

Misdirection: *"I hate to see misled people work hard in the gym, only to have their results ruined by eating the wrong foods."* – John Parrillo

4
SIZZLING
SUPPLEMENTS

The impact of good nutrition on building muscle (both direct and indirect) can be magnified with the use of supplements. The dictionary defines *supplement* as "something that completes, or an addition to." Supplements both complete and add to the effect nutrition has on the physique. Supplements are vital to producing maximum results. If you look at the dietary intake of almost any top professional, you will observe the frequent use of supplements. Supplementation provides a certain unique boost to body development.

No Magic Potion

One of the most important aspects to realize is that they are "supplements" – they supplement something else. That something else is food. Food is what a hungry body needs. The whole of a food makes up more than just the sum of its parts (supplementation makes use of some of those parts). Elements of foods are still being discovered. There continues to be an x factor, elements and especially the interaction of different elements in food that research has not yet grasped. The body best digests food in its natural state.

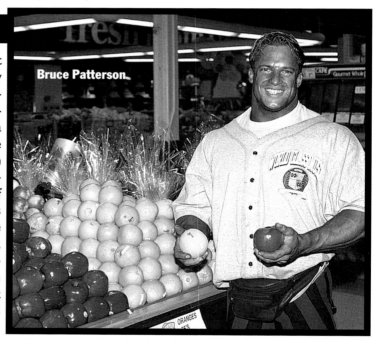

Bruce Patterson

Supplements are not more important than food and should not be expected to take the place of the central role of a sound intake of solid, natural food. Many novice bodybuilders look to supplements to be some magic potion, some key ingredient that will supernaturally transform the physique into instant mounds of rock-hard muscle. That just won't happen. Supplements are not magic – they are the result of scientific means to isolate and maximize the use of certain nutrients and associated elements. They do provide many benefits – benefits often unique to the bodybuilding community. There are dozens of supplement companies out there – it's a major money-making industry. Some products work well, others are so-so, and some don't do a thing. It can be hard to sort through the hype to find what does and does not enhance the

Supplements are not magic. No single element, dietary or otherwise, will instantaneously transform a soft physique into rock-hard muscle.

musclebuilding process. This chapter will provide a guide to what works in the area of supplements for building the body, and how to avoid spending hard-earned money on something that won't do a thing for you, or worse, may even harm the body.

Direct & Indirect Effect

Many novice trainers look for the fast and easy path to a powerful physique. If it is fast and easy, most likely it won't be effective! A powerful and muscular physique is the result of several factors coming together over time. Certainly supplementation can help make the process happen faster, but no single supplement is the answer. Along these lines, you must recognize the interplay between many nutrients and substances. You run up a red flag that shows you are a novice if you place all your hopes in one single *magic pill* to do the trick and give you gigantic muscle in one fell swoop. That won't happen. If you rely on a supplement to carry the entire load of changing your physique, and changing it right now, you will lose both money and time.

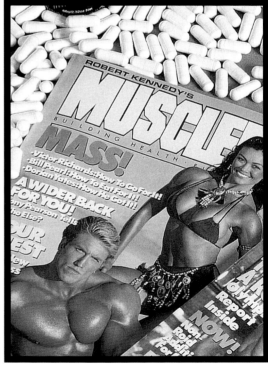

What happens next is predictable. Those who hold such beliefs become discouraged and soon quit. To avoid this common mistake, look to the full spectrum of training for the answers. Realize that supplementation, while not the central pillar, is in fact one of the supporting beams of the muscle-making process.

A bodybuilding columnist recently lamented the fact that a novice had written him asking why he had recommended some supplement that was more for the health of the body than specifically for building muscle size. This novice was missing the point. The body works as a unit. If one component is dragging the immune system down, the muscle growth factor will not be given priority. For muscle to grow, all systems must be good to go, and

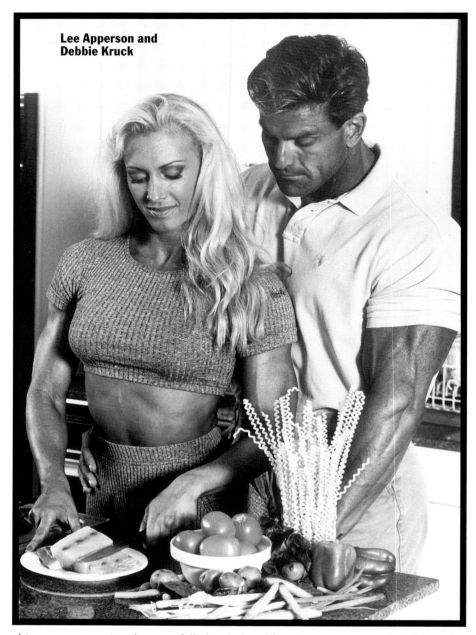

Lee Apperson and
Debbie Kruck

this means ensuring they are fully loaded and functioning as intended. Often the best way to encourage muscle growth through supplementation is indirectly. If the body is up and running as it should be, then it is free to grant priority to muscle growth. By the way, beyond the initial growing phase through late adolescence, muscle growth is not a priority of the body. Its priorities are more basic – keeping the immune system strong, healing the body from illness, etc. Ignore this point to your own detriment.

Necessity of Supplementation

If regular food is so great, why supplement your diet? There are several reasons to make supplementation a regular habit. First, food preparation in modern culture removes many of the nutrients from what we eat. Even as a bodybuilder taking care to eat nutritiously, you often cannot avoid this factor. The more refined the food, the less substantial nutrients it will provide. Almost everything is becoming more refined. Read the list of ingedients on the label of the food you purchase. More than likely it is full of additives, and lacking any real nutritional value. Even the cooking process causes loss of nutrients. The same is particularly true for fast foods and restaurant meals. As part of your own social community, it is hard to avoid dining out on occasion. Dining out is the fastest growing trend in the food world, second to ordering a pizza to eat at home in front of the television! Add to this predicament the stress of daily life, environmental pollution, and a host of other contributing factors, and the need for supplementation becomes readily apparent. Consider the fact that some soils are deficient in nutrients such as chromium. These issues apply to everyone, not just the bodybuilder. It is a good idea for everyone to incorporate some level of supplementation.

> *Often the best way to benefit muscle growth through supplementation is indirectly.*

Specific Supplementation

Bodybuilders need specific supplementation for they have unique needs since the pursuit of adding skeletal muscle beyond the norm is unique – even among other athletes. They require more protein. Getting that extra protein through more meals can be a problem due to the extra calories, carbs and fat that naturally come in a full meal. A supplement in the form of protein powder can address that problem directly, providing the protein without the added 500 calories that a meal would bring. Time is another consideration. Who has time to stop and make a full meal several times every day. A protein powder shake or meal-replacement drink or bar fits the need almost perfectly.

Other considerations include the higher nutrient level needed for the demanding workouts with heavy iron. The very *nature* of building muscle calls for special supplementation because the body is being pushed to expand beyond the normal parameters of the sedentary masses. Under stress the body needs more of the nutrients, but without all the associated calories in regular food. Again supplementation fits the bill. A bodybuilder has not only the daily stress of work, relationships, the environment, but also the demands of the gym. Supplementation is a great tool. It provides quick nutrient intake in specific amounts for specific needs.

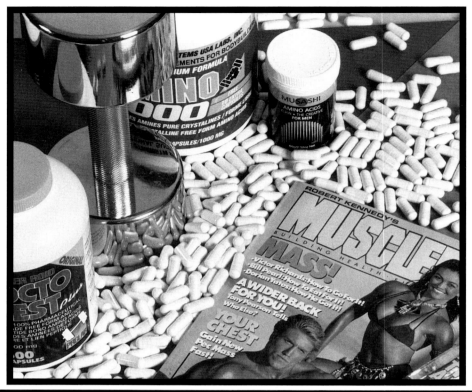

Where Do You Start?

Do you just run out and buy whatever supplements are on sale? Or whichever has the flashiest ad campaign in the various muscle magazines? Go that route and you will quickly be relieved of your money. Supplements are not cheap, so put your money where it counts. Choose a specific target. Find what the body needs most and what works.

Generally the best time to take a supplement is along with or right after a meal. Taking some supplements on an empty stomach (particularly vitamins) can cause minor discomfort in the stomach. If you must take a supplement between meals, eat something solid with it – a cracker, rice cake, etc. Some types of supplements work best separately, or act as their own meal (protein shakes, meal replacements), but the general rule is to take supplements (particularly those in tablet form) with or just after a meal.

Multivitamin/Mineral

Start your supplementation with a multivitamin/mineral to cover the bases in areas you may be lacking. Take the multivitamin at least five times a week (give your body two days off on weekends). If possible, go with the powdered form as this can be added easily to a protein or meal-replacement shake. When choosing to buy a multi, read the label carefully and make sure you're getting at least 50 percent of the RDA for all the vitamins and minerals. Most will provide 100 percent or more of the RDA of just the popular vitamins and some minerals, but skimp on some of the less popular but still vital minerals. Demand more out of your multi and get *at least* 50 percent coverage on everything, with 100 percent coverage on the popular vitamins and minerals. If you can find a multi that lists everything at 100 percent or more of the RDA, go with that one. All are equally significant in meeting the needs of the human body. You will pay more for the natural source-based multis, but they are certainly better than synthetic.

Protein Powders

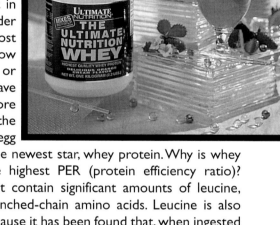

Over the years protein has probably been the most popular supplement in the bodybuilding community. The powder form allows for the addition of almost pure protein to the diet, with a low calorie/carb base. Most are nonfat or low-fat as well. Protein powders have evolved over time and are even more effective now than earlier. Some of the popular mixes are milk protein, egg protein, milk and egg protein, and the newest star, whey protein. Why is whey such a favorite when egg has the highest PER (protein efficiency ratio)? Unfortunately egg protein does not contain significant amounts of leucine, which is one of the most vital branched-chain amino acids. Leucine is also singled out here in Chapter Four because it has been found that, when ingested within 15 minutes of the completion of a workout, the leucine appears to quick-start the protein rebuilding process — allowing the muscle to recover more quickly. Leucine is used up by the body during exercise. Avery's *Almanac* notes: "For an athlete whose protein intake is marginal, this (lack of leucine) could be a negative factor in recuperation and growth." It is interesting to note that whey protein has twice as much leucine as egg protein.

There is a large and growing body of information supporting the supremacy of whey protein. Whey protein is known to benefit the immune system (which is vital for full body functioning). Whey protein is the strongest in the area of the important branched-chain amino acids. Whey is also known to

Whey protein is the strongest in the area of the important branched-chain amino acids.

mix up well (although some of the early versions a few years ago went down rough). Whey is a good choice for protein powder supplementation.

Although egg protein is not as plentiful in leucine, it does have a host of other beneficial properties which make it a close second to whey. Egg is a top-level protein choice. One benefit for those who struggle in this area is that most versions are lactose free. Egg protein is often offered in combination with milk protein.

Milk proteins have been putting muscle on bodybuilders for years. Although surpassed in level of protein quality by the egg and whey combination, milk protein (the main type is casein, a cousin of whey) does provide good amounts of glutamine.

Soy protein is all the rage once again. Many years ago soy was touted as a great protein source. It does not have as complete a range of the essential amino acids as do whey and egg protein. After all, soy is a vegetable. Soy is probably the best protein for women due to the estrogenic effect. Soy protein's ability to be mixed and taste has improved significantly since the early years.

Dry milk is the poor man's choice for adding protein to the diet. Powdered milk contains a good deal of fat-free protein which can be mixed in water or milk and blended with yogurt and/or another flavoring such as vanilla or honey to create a very good protein supplement at a minimal cost. Although not as high-tech as the latest commercial blends, this protein shake will support muscle growth.

Meal Replacements

Meal replacement mixes are somewhat similar to protein powders except the meal replacement usually contains a broader range of nutrients. In addition to the protein, quality carbs and fats are added as well as vitamins, minerals, and other related elements. Many of the top bodybuilders now incorporate meal replacement bars or shakes in their weekly menus. Meal replacements come in handy time-wise and since they are more complete than the protein powders, allow for longer bridges between solid food meals. *Avery's Almanac* points out several situations where meal-replacement powders can be very beneficial:
• as a precompetition, postcompetition or postworkout meal,
  or as a regular meal in the off-season
• to maintain bodyweight
• to lose weight
• as a high-energy snack
• to increase lean body mass

The meal replacement can take the place of a regular meal if you're trying to lose weight. It can be added between meals to help you gain weight, or used for postworkout refueling.

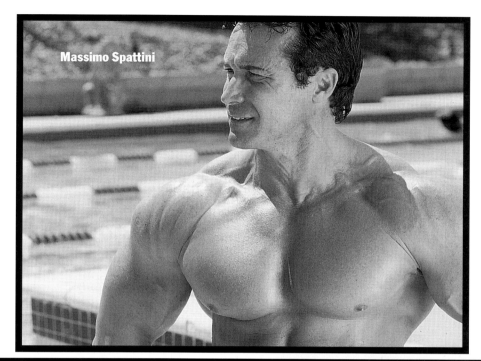

Massimo Spattini

Supplement Spotlight

So far the review of supplements has been broad – multivitamin/minerals, protein powders and meal replacement mixes. You can also benefit by increasing the intake of certain individual nutrients. You can accomplish that by eating more regular foods, but you may find it easier to add the nutrients to your daily intake in supplement form – tablet, liquid or powder.

Vital Vitamin C

Arguably the most popular supplement of all, vitamin C is also one of the most neglected substances by bodybuilders. If you are looking to build up your muscles, chances are you wouldn't think of turning to vitamin C.

This nutrient gained fame before it was ever specifically identified as a vitamin. English sailors in the late 18th century depended on citrus fruit to prevent the painful problems of scurvy. Sailors who ate limes avoided the disease. The power of vitamin C became official in 1932 and gained fame as research identified it as the substance that cured scurvy. Vitamin C gained even more press a few decades later when Linus Pauling, two-time Nobel laureate and the world's foremost vitamin C proponent, started digging into the capabilities of this fascinating nutrient. His *Vitamin C and the Common Cold* took the world by storm and since then almost every mother pumps her child full of vitamin C during the cold and flu season.

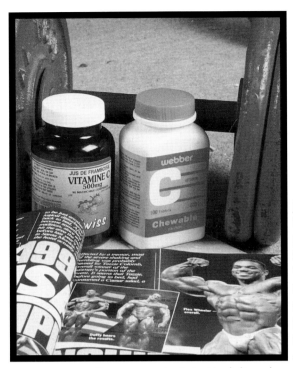

Vitamin C is an important part of the body's defense against muscle damage from exercise.

Vitamin C, however, is more than just a cold remedy. This nutrient is involved in more than 300 biological processes within the body. This vitamin is one of the most powerful elements. Vitamin C deficiency can lead to slower healing of wounds, increased suscepibility to infections, as well as male infertility and increased genetic damage to sperm cells (which may lead to birth defects). Vitamin C deficiency may also contribute to gastrointestinal disorders and rheumatoid arthritis.

Surprisingly, many people overlook the importance of this vitamin — and that is especially unfortunate for those who work out. While not as glamorous as the latest line of supplements such as creatine or whey protein, vitamin C is a worthwhile training aid. Supplement guru Bill Phillips discovered in a survey that very few hardcore fitness and bodybuilding trainers even take vitamin C regularly. That is, the group of people who probably need the nutrient the most are neglecting to take it. Vitamin C has made the top list in Phillips's famous annual supplement review even though it is not a glamour nutrient (famous yes, glamorous no). He points to research that suggests this vitamin may do more than just act as an antioxidant — it may help improve the overall ratio of testosterone to cortisol as well as help contractile tension (for strength) and assist the tendons and ligaments. Dr. Michael Colgan also points out (in his *Colgan Chronicals*) that vitamin C reduces cortisol levels. For those reasons and more, Phillips favors strong intake. A recent article in *Physical* magazine also stated vitamin C has been shown to suppress levels of the muscle-wasting hormone cortisol. That decrease is of tremendous benefit to the bodybuilder in producing muscle growth.

If you are looking to get the most out of your training, particularly on a consistent basis, make sure you don't overlook the benefits of this nutrient. Vitamin C is a vital nutritional tool for helping the body to recover: "Antioxidants such as vitamins C and E are an important part of the body's defense against muscle damage from exercise. Strenuous exercise increases the body's production of free radicals, which, in turn, can cause muscle damage which manifests itself as swollen or painful muscles. While exercise increases the body's natural level of defense against free radicals, athletes who are doing *intense training* may benefit from the addition of antioxidant supplements to their diets." – From "The role of antioxidant vitamins and enzymes in the prevention of exercise-induced muscle damage." *Sports Med* 1996;21(3):213-38.

Vitamin C helps your body recover from strenuous workouts (resistance training and cardiovascular/aerobic training) and more. If you care about your long-term health you don't want to overlook vitamin C (ascorbic acid), a water-soluble vitamin and one powerful antioxidant. C is needed to make collagen for muscles and blood vessels. It is important for healing wounds and acts as a natural antihistamine. This important vitamin helps the body fight viruses as well. A study in the *Journal of Epidemiology* (May 1992) was reported to show that people who have high blood levels of vitamin C live six years longer than those with lower blood levels. In doses of approximately one gram daily, vitamin C has also been shown to help protect the body against LDL (the bad type of cholesterol), says the *American Journal of Clinical Nutrition*.

The role of vitamin C and collagen should be of particular interest to those who train with weights in an effort to increase muscularity. In fact the main role of vitamin C is not to fight colds, but to manufacture collagen. According to Linus Pauling, the versatility of vitamin C in illness prevention arises from its role in the manufacture of collagen, the protein that gives shape to connective tissues and strength to skin and blood vessels. Collagen is the protein that forms the basis of connective tissue (the most abundant tissue in the body). Connective tissue acts as a cementing substance between cells. Collagen protects and helps support the muscles, bones, joints and more, as well as promotes healing of wounds, fractures and bruises. All of these elements are important for those who stimulate the body to high levels of conditioning via repeated workouts. Even the ability to fight viruses (as noted in *J Vit Nutr Res Supplement)* is beneficial to those who train frequently and need to keep the body in top working condition.

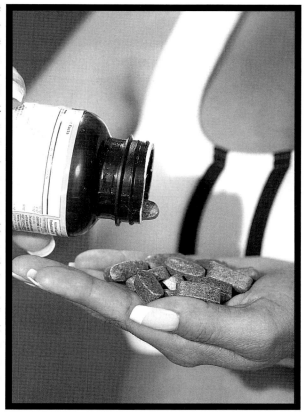

The natural source of vitamin C is not limited to oranges and citrus fruits. Tasty foods such as strawberries and kiwi fruit are high in C. So are red peppers, acerola berries, broccoli, parsley, currants, rose hips and even brussel sprouts. Consider taking this vitamin tablet if you eat on the run frequently and are not able to get this vital nutrient from natural sources. The US Recommended Daily Amount (RDA) for vitamin C is 60 milligrams. However, researchers at the National Institutes of Health recommend that the RDA for vitamin C be raised to 200 mg per day. Dr. Michael Colgan states "For athletes we recommend between 3000 and 6000 mg per day of vitamin C." *(Colgan Chronicles)* Linus Pauling is an advocate of higher intake of the vitamin. Body tissue stores of vitamin C are small and easily saturated, with any excess removed within two to three hours.

A word of caution on increasing the intake of vitamin C – people taking anticlotting medications may unwittingly abolish the effect if they take massive doses of vitamin C *(Understanding Nutrition, Whitney, Rolfes)*. Vitamin C interferes with anticoagulants such as heparin and coumadin. Also, those who have a tendency toward gout or genetic abnormality that alters vitamin C breakdown are prone to kidney stones if they take large doses of C *(Ibid)*.

Don't overlook the importance of this vitamin as a dietary aid to realizing the best from your body. This is not just another celebrity vitamin – it is a vital tool for keeping your body in top condition. Vitamin C can definitely boost your musclebuilding efforts.

Antioxidants

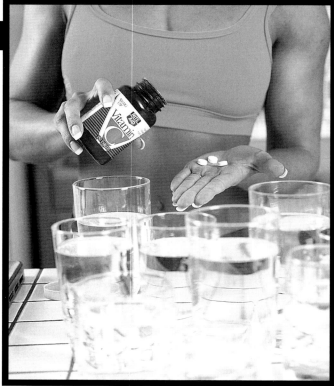

A group of vitamins called *antioxidants* (primarily A, C, E and sometimes zinc) have received a lot of press over the past few years, primarily in relation to heart health. The following overview comes from the American Heart Association Science Advisory:

"Considerable evidence now suggests that oxidants are involved in the development and clinical expression of coronary heart disease, and that anti-oxidants may contribute to disease resistance. Consistent with this view, epidemiological evidence indicates that greater antioxidant intake is associated with lower disease risk. Although this increased antioxidant intake generally has involved increased consumption of antioxidant-rich foods, some obser-

"You only get one body, so you must treat it with respect."
– Kim Lyons

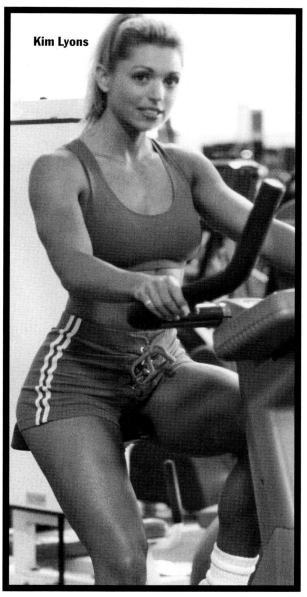

Kim Lyons

vational studies have suggested the importance of levels of vitamin C intake achievable only by supplementation. There is currently no such evidence from primary prevention trials, but results from secondary prevention trials have shown beneficial effects of vitamin C supplements on the duration of some diseases.

"In contrast, trials directly addressing the effect of beta-carotene supplementation have not shown beneficial effects, and some have suggested deleterious effects, particularly in high-risk population subgroups. In view of these findings, the most prudent and scientifically supportable recommendation for the general population is to consume a balanced diet with emphasis on antioxidant-rich fruits and vegetables and whole grains. This advice, which is consistent with the current dietary guidelines of the American Heart Association, considers the role of the total diet in influencing disease risk. Although diet alone may not provide the levels of vitamin E intake that have been associated with the lowest risk in a few observational studies, the absence of efficacy and safety data from randomized trials precludes the establishment of population-wide recommendations regarding vitamin E supplementation. In the case of secondary prevention [protection of people who are known to have coronary artery disease], the results from clinical trials of vitamin C have been encouraging, and if further studies confirm these findings, consideration of the merits of vitamin E supplementation in individuals with cardiovascular disease would be warranted."

The best source of antioxidants is regular food. The backup, of course, is supplementation. Some research from the University of California suggests athletes can reduce their muscle cell damage from exercise by taking antioxidants. Research from Penn State University has indicated that vitamin E (the study utilized supplementation) is quite beneficial for muscle recovery. An exciting new era in the area of antioxidant supplementation is just beginning. Igene Biotechnology's marketing company, ProBio Nutraceuticals, recently introduced a formulated natural astaxanthin from Igene as a new superantioxidant, AstaBioCare®, into the North American dietary supplement market. What's that? *www.astaxanthin.org* notes:

"Astaxanthin, a naturally occurring carotenoid pigment, is a powerful biological antioxidant. Astaxanthin exhibits strong free radical scavenging activity and protects against lipid peroxidation and oxidative damage of LDL cholesterol, cell membranes, cells and tissues. As astaxanthin is one of the most potent and bio-active biological antioxidants found in nature, this abundance of research on antioxidants suggests a number of potential roles of astaxanthin for human health. Additional benefits could also result from astaxanthin properties other than its well-known antioxidant power."

Astaxanthin has been the focus of a large and growing number of peer-reviewed scientific publications lately. Watch for further developments on this horizon.

King Chromium

Chromium is a mineral that plays a vital role in the diet because it stimulates the activity of enzymes involved in the metabolism of glucose for energy and the synthesis of fatty acids and cholesterol. Chromium appears to increase the effectiveness of insulin and its ability to handle glucose, preventing hypoglycemia (too much insulin) or diabetes (too little insulin) – as noted in the *Nutrition Almanac*. Getting adequate chromium is very important, particularly if you live in the United States where the soil is generally lacking in chromium. The modern diet seems to supply a lot of the necessary minerals – except chromium. Scientists at the United States Department of Agriculture (USDA) have pointed out that most people are not getting adequate chromium in their diets. The problem has existed for some time and is expanding due to the increasing reliance on highly processed refined foods, which are high in sugar and fat. According to USDA studies, nine out of ten Americans get less than 50 micrograms of chromium daily as compared to the 50 to 200 micrograms recommended by the National Academy of Sciences (Nutrition 21). That's significant. It means 90 percent of the population is not getting enough of this powerful mineral. That includes bodybuilders. Obtaining sufficient chromium intake is important for both energy flow and other functions.

In the *International Journal of Sport Nutrition* (1993;3:117-122), Gary Evans, PhD describes a study in which he gave chromium supplements to six men and six women enrolled in a weekly aerobics class. Lean body mass in the women taking 200 mcg chromium picolinate daily increased by about 4 pounds compared to just over 1 pound among those taking an equal amount of chromium nicotinate. Lean body mass among the men taking chromium picolinate increased by 4.6 pounds compared to 1.5 pounds among those taking the other form of the mineral. Chromium is advantageous for the fully functioning physique and plays an integral role in controlling energy levels. Don't overlook the importance of chromium, which is found in abundance in brewer's yeast. But listen up – if you are on medication for control of your blood sugar, make sure to check with your doctor before using chromium due to blood sugar reactions.

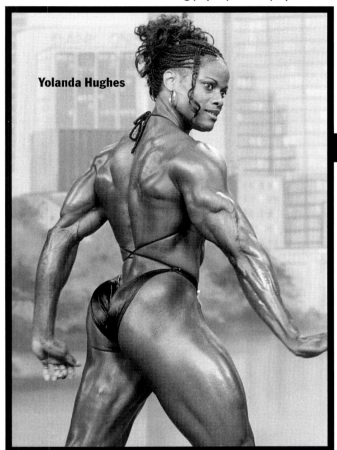

Yolanda Hughes

Brewer's Yeast

Brewer's yeast is not a single mineral, but does contain many minerals and vitamins. Brewer's yeast is simply the top superfood on the market. It has more protein than a sirloin steak, liver or powdered milk. To top it off, this excellent food source contains no fat. When you obtain quality protein, fat is usually part of the package. Not so with brewer's yeast. It has a super protein-to-fat ratio. The amino acid profile is broad also, as brewer's yeast protein comes from 16 amino acids. Does it contain leucine? Yes. Brewer's yeast is a veritable one-a-day vitamin in itself. Most food items contain just a few vitamins; brewer's yeast contains 17. That is incredible for a single food source.

The most potent supplement is definitely brewer's yeast: high protein, fiber, no fat, 16 amino acids, 17 vitamins, 14 minerals, chromium, nucleic acids – virtually a complete food.

But wait, there's more. Brewer's yeast also contains 14 minerals. It is one of the premium sources of nucleic acids (RNA-DNA) which are important in keeping the body immune to degenerative disease *(Nutrition Amanac)*, slowing down the aging process, and recharging worn out cells (Gironda). Brewer's yeast is a potent source for enzyme-producing agents. Add to this the fact that this substance is one of the top natural sources of chromium. Furthermore, brewer's yeast is a strong source of fiber. One serving provides six grams. One serving of brewer's yeast also contains the suggested daily amount of chromium.

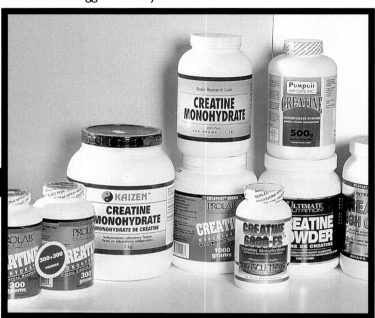

If you can afford only one supplement, consider making it this one. Yes, it has been around for a long time; no, nothing has topped it as a super food supplement yet. For a better flavor use the "debittered" form of brewer's yeast.

Creatine

You would almost have to be a hermit to not have heard of this stuff. Everyone is using it. From football players to baseball, and probably even golfers, creatine was the big star of the mid to late '90s. Advanced formulas are now the rage. Creatine is a substance that the body manufactures, and it can also be obtained through food sources. This past decade it has become available in supplement form. The Web site *www.nutritionsupplements.com* notes that creatine is a compound your body forms on its own in the amount of about 2 mg per day. This small quantity does not cause any problems with kidney stones and the like. However, when taking creatine supplements in the amounts advised by bodybuilders and salespeople, usually around 10 to 20 mg per day, you have an increased risk of developing kidney stones because of the insolubility that is in such saturated amounts. Creatine works to give you excess energy (beyond what is normal) so you can work out longer and develop more muscle. It does this by acting as a supplement ATP. Your body can then regenerate its ATP supply and you still have the energy to work out. This prevents you from going anaerobic and developing lactic acid buildup.

Creatine has been found to increase body size. *Avery's Almanac* states scientific research verifies that creatine increases muscle strength and power, promotes significant increases in lean body mass and muscle without a

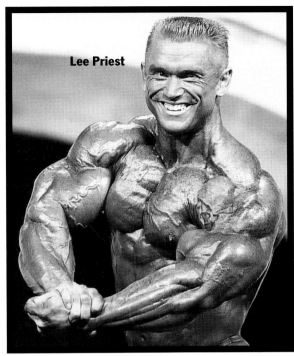
Lee Priest

corresponding gain in bodyfat, improves performance during short-term high-intensity exercise, hastens recovery between high-intensity resistance-training workouts, may reduce fatigue by decreasing the lactic acid buildup, may increase the anaerobic threshold, and allows for more intense training. That's powerful incentive for almost anyone to try creatine. What must be factored into the equation is, there is also an ongoing debate on whether or not creatine has a nasty effect on the kidneys.

The potential long-term hazards are mostly unknown. Use of this substance is quite high, even among the young. Dr. Jordan D. Metzl, a specialist in sports medicine at New York's Hospital for Special Surgery, presented a study at the combined annual meeting of the Pediatric Academic Societies and the American Academy of Pediatrics. The study revealed that, among students in 12th grade, 44 percent admitted to creatine use. Reuters Health reported that two youngsters are known to have suffered kidney failure in the last three years after taking creatine.

Manufacturers are constantly working on upgrading this product. Manufacturer of Creatine Serum, *www.creatine.com,* points out: Creatine powder is highly insoluble, so athletes must ingest large amounts in order to have any reach their muscles. These excess amounts of creatine powder precipitate out into the liver and kidneys, creating the potential of long-term side effects. But because Creatine Serum is so highly soluble, it reaches the muscles quickly and safely, bypassing the digestive system altogether. Athletes need to use only a very small amount of it to achieve effective results. There is no wastage or buildup in the organs.

Avery's Almanac features several articles touting the benefits of creatine intake, including an article in *Medicine and Science in Sports and Exercise* on a study which noted that creatine increased gains in muscle mass. Another article in *CDC Morbidity* and *Mortality Weekly Report* found that three deaths originally thought to have some link to creatine intake were instead due to other factors. Please note that long-term side effects are still up in the air since use of creatine by the mainstream athletic community as a whole is only recent. Caffeine blocks creatine; creatine's a diuretic, meaning that drinking it can lead to dehydration, so take plenty of water if you do use creatine. The US RDA is 2 grams per day.

Some recommend a loading phase. If you decide to use creatine, start off with small amounts and watch the way your body responds – not only your muscles, but also your kidneys.

Desiccated Liver

Yes, I know Bill Phillips doesn't rank it very high in his supplement review. However, desiccated liver is another superfood. It was a favorite supplement recommended by the late Vince Gironda. Why? Desiccated liver is four times as potent as raw liver. It has a high protein content and its net protein utilization is high (80 percent), which is equivalent to fish, better than meat or chicken, and far ahead of soy. Desiccated liver is a blood-builder, contains nucleic acids, iron, and a full spectrum of B vitamins. It also is a good source of calcium, copper, phosphorous, and vitamins A, C and D. It has a naturally occurring amino profile.

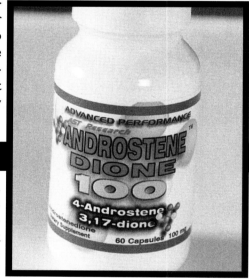

Vince Gironda pointed out that desiccated liver contains a growth factor as well as an antiestrogen to keep testosterone levels high in the male bodybuilder. He advised taking several tablets interspersed throughout the day (two per meal) and gradually increasing the amount taken.

Androstenedione

Androstenedione, known as andro, was once almost as popular as creatine. Probably the most well-known user is home run king Mark McGwire, most likely because it is not banned by the Major Baseball League. It is banned, however, by the NFL, the NCAA, and the International Olympic Committee. Add to that the NBA:

Androstenedione Added to NBA List of Banned Substances

New York (March 30, 2000) XINHUA – Androstenedione has been added to the list of drugs banned by the National Basketball Association. Androstenedione, a performance-enhancing drug taken by US major league baseball's Mark McGwire when he hit a record 70 home runs in 1988, is banned by most sports and the Olympics, but not by baseball. Yesterday the NBA said the NBA-NBPA Players Association Prohibited Substances Committee added androstenedione and eight other substances to the list of steroids banned by the NBA-NBPA Anti-Drug Agreement.

These governing bodies view it as an enhancement that falls out of the parameters of acceptable use, considering it similar to steroids.

The first few versions of a supplement are sometimes not as effective or safe as later upgrades.

Young Again online notes andro is a hormone found in all animals as well as some plants. It is a metabolite of DHEA that serves as a direct precurser of testosterone, the principal male sex hormone. Androstenedione is produced in the gonads and adrenal glands and is required for the growth and maturation of the male sex organs.

For what reasons do people take andro? The belief is that andro raises testosterone levels. The hope is that this will translate into gains in muscle size and/or benefits in performance. Andro was reported to have been used by the East German Olympic Team to enhance athletic performance by increasing testosterone levels. However, the substance reportedly does not stay in the bloodstream very long, and large amounts of andro are needed to bring about the required effect.

As with creatine, there are serious health concerns associated with androstenedione. Androstenedione is also relatively new to the consumer market. Remember, the early bird gets the worm, but the second mouse gets the cheese. That thought is helpful when considering whether or not to try something before adequate long-term studies have been conducted on the side effects. Let someone else be the guinea pig for the newer supplements on the market until enough testing has been done to assess both the benefits of the supplement and any side effects of concern. The first few versions of a supplement are sometimes not as effective or safe as later upgrades.

The main concern associated with using andro is the health of the prostate. One study in *Avery's Almanac* noted data that suggested andro could influence latent forms of prostate cancer. However, *JAMA (Journal of the American Medical Association),* looked into the use of andro and didn't find much wrong with it. An online critique of the *JAMA* findings noted: The *JAMA*

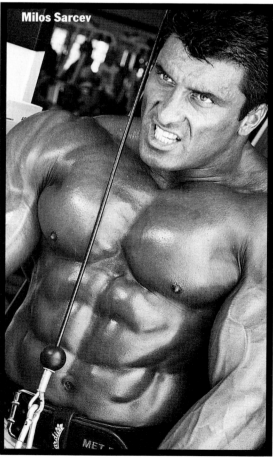

Milos Sarcev

investigators found androstenedione to be safe, but warn that this finding doesn't rule out an adverse reaction from sustained use. The *JAMA* authors speculate about potential downsides of oral use, and these concerns were picked up in press reports. Extraneous inferences to potential heart disease, pancreatic and prostate cancer, and liver malfunction detracted from an otherwise sound study.

The main concern seemed to be the long-term effects of andro intake. Owen Fonorow's overview of the study, "*JAMA* Study on Androstenedione – A Critique" points out: The *JAMA* commentary discusses the Anabolic Steroid Control Act of 1990 and notes testosterone and a number of derivatives as Schedule III drugs under the Controlled Substance Act. Since androstenedione is not specifically mentioned, it can only be banned if the following criteria are met: 1) the substance must have a molecular structure related to testosterone, 2) the substance must have a pharmacology related to testosterone, 3) the

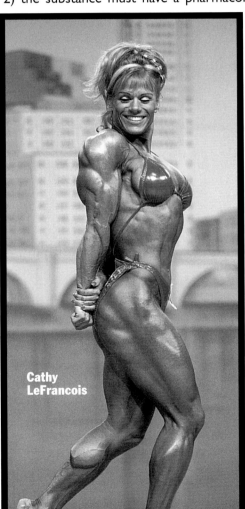

Cathy
LeFrancois

substance cannot be an estrogen, progestin or corticosteroid, and 4) the substance must promote muscle growth. In its commentary on the study, the *JAMA* editor admits that the King et al. study data show that androstenedione does not meet the fourth criterion (that is, it does not promote muscle growth).

Fonorow makes this point: "The authors classify androstenedione as a "weak anabolic steroid," yet the AMA would still like to see this substance off the market. They seem to want it both ways. The substance is ineffective but should be removed from the market. Which is it?"

The use of andro in the general public arena is still in its infancy (there have been only a few major studies conducted to date). The best approach is to give researchers more time before making a decision on whether or not to try it. Long-term side effects of supplement substance use can be pronounced. Remember, the second mouse gets the cheese – so don't be first.

Wheat Germ

Wheat germ can be classified as either a food or a supplement. The wheat germ itself is used as a cereal; the oil is often sold in capsules or liquid form as a supplement. Wheat germ qualifies as a "superfood" due to its many potent positive qualities. Wheat germ oil is strong in unsaturated fatty acids, iron, vitamins A, B and E, and folic acid. Wheat germ also contains good amounts of zinc, phosphorus, magnesium and potassium. Gironda noted its antistress and endurance factors. Wheat germ in the regular form has good amounts of fiber as well. Four tablespoons of wheat germ in the cereal form provide 8 grams of protein, 4 grams of fiber, only 2 grams of fat (but the good type, polyunsaturated), no cholesterol, no sodium, 8 percent of the daily requirement of potassium, 20 percent of the RDA for zinc, mostly complex carbs, and only 100 calories. That is a super nutritional profile!

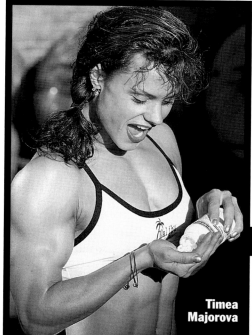

Timea Majorova

The best supplements contain a variety of strong nutrients and associated factors (such as fiber). The more you are forced to split your supplementation up into single areas the more expensive it becomes. You lose some of the natural interplay between nutrients as well. Since wheat germ contains a host of positive nutrient factors in a single source, it is a top food supplement choice. Use it on your cereal, or take the oil in capsule or bottled form. The cereal form is probably the best due to the fiber content.

Ephedrine/Ephedra

Ephedrine, also known as ephedra, has been the darling of the weight-loss groupies for the past decade or so. Ephedrine goes under many names, such as ma huang and various street names. Again, controversy swirls around the use of this supplementary substance.

Ephedrine is primarily prized for its bodyfat-burning effects, but it is not a single-response substance. Taking ephedrine provides other results as well. *Encyclopedia.com* lists this description: "ephedrine – mild, slow-acting drug used to treat moderate attacks of bronchial asthma and to relieve nasal congestion from hay fever or infection of the upper respiratory tract. Nonaddictive, ephedrine may cause insomnia and restlessness."

The *ephedrine-ephedra.com* site lists a more complete description of this substance: What is ephedrine, ephedra ... ma huang? These terms refer to the same substance derived from the plant *ephedra*. (There are many common names for these evergreen plants, including squaw tea and Mormon tea.) Ephedra is a shrub-like plant found in desert regions of Central Asia and other parts of the world. The dried greens of the plant are used medicinally. Ephedra is a stimulant that contains the herbal form of ephedrine, an FDA-regulated drug found in over-the-counter asthma medications. In the United States ephedra and ephedrine are sold in health-food stores under a number of brand names. Ephedrine is widely used for weight loss, as an energy booster, and to enhance athletic performance. These products often contain other stimulants such as caffeine, which may have synergistic effects and increase the potential for adverse effects. Ephedra is often touted as the "herbal fen-phen."

One of Bill Phillips's *Supplement Review* articles notes that originally the sale of ephedrine was unrestricted, but due to a few reported deaths allegedly attributed to ephedrine, the sale of the this herb derivative has become restricted. Consider this health news blurb: The Food and Drug Administration continues to duke it out with industry over the safety of the dietary supplement ephedra. The *Wall Street Journal* quoted Lori Love of the FDA with this statement: "Adverse effects can be predicted and should be anticipated if consumers continue to use these (ephedra-based) products." Industry experts contend that the studies referred to by the government lack key data and detail. The industry points to the millions of people who have used the supplements without adverse reactions. The burden of proof lies with the government, according to current law.

Massimo Spattini, Jennifer Stimac and Michelle Mann

And the government continues to go after ephedrine – this substance could become fully regulated in the near future. Why? The *ephedrine-ephedra.com* site online states, "The FDA believe ephedra may be related to more than 50 deaths. Most of the serious injuries involve high blood pressure that can cause bleeding in the brain, stroke or heart attack."

Ephedrine has caused problems for some people. Many have taken it without adverse reactions. If you choose to use this substance, do so in low doses and make sure to carefully monitor your body's reactions.

Alfalfa

Here is a supplement without a lot of controversy or negative press dogging it. Alfalfa is known as the father of all foods and is one of nature's richest sources of crucial nutrients. Alfalfa contains an abundant supply of important vitamins, minerals and enzymes. It is the strongest detoxicant of any food and is the best source of calcium around – even better than milk. Alfalfa contains the essential amino acids and is a good source of protein. Taking a few tablets a day after meals can benefit the body in many ways.

An Extra Edge

Supplementation can provide your body with an extra edge in gaining muscle and burning off fat to reveal that muscle. Supplements are not magic beans – they won't bring about huge gains overnight. However, they can help the muscle growth process. Your basic minimum supplements used should be multi- vitamin/minerals, protein powders and meal replacements. Brewer's yeast is also a mainstay of any good program. Beyond this, there are hundreds of other supplements available. You will want to try some to see if they give your body a boost. Do not take massive doses of any product; however, do be consistent in the supplement intake and give the product time to work. Remember, good results are not instantaneous.

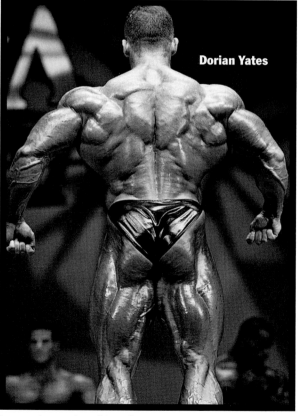

Dorian Yates

• Many supplements can help pro-mote muscle growth as well as fat loss.
• Supplements don't work magic. They won't bring about instant results.
• Supplements need time to work. Be consistent in taking them.
• All supplements do not work. Don't hesitate to discard a supplement if you are not getting results after a reasonable period of time.
• Some supplements may have harmful side effects. Carefully monitor your body's reactions to any supplement, and study up on any substance you plan on taking.

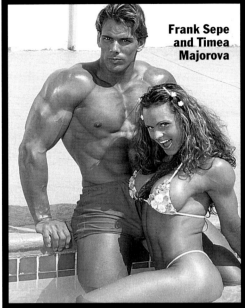

Frank Sepe and Timea Majorova

Thoughts From the Pros on Supplements

Diet comes first: *"Supplementation is not nearly as important as eating a well-balanced and nutritious diet."* – Dorian Yates

On vitamin/mineral intake: *"Vitamins are organic substances and should be consumed with food and minerals for best absorption. The body works on a 24-hour cycle. Your cells don't sleep when you do, nor can they function without a continuous supply of oxygen and nutrients. For best results with vitamin and mineral supplements, space them throughout the day and take them after meals. If that's not practical, take half after breakfast and half after dinner. If you must take them all at once, do it after your largest meal."* – Peter Nielsen

Multivitamin/mineral: *"No athlete should go without a multivitamin/mineral supplement."* – Lee Labrada

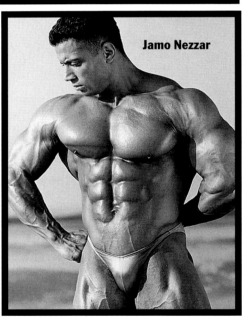

Jamo Nezzar

Supplements: *"I try to eat a lot of whole, unprocessed foods, but take supplements as needed. I've had a lot of success with MET-Rx products."* – Mark Dugdale, Mr. Seattle

Diet and supplements: *"Start eating correctly when you begin your program. Diet is the key to losing weight. Remember, training and diet go hand in hand. I don't disagree with taking supplements or vitamins – as long as it's in moderation."* – Frank Sepe

Off-season supplementation: *"I do not tend to use too many supplements during the off-season. I take vitamin C in large quantities and use a good multivitamin. I really rate glutamine. Depending upon your financial situation, use it as often as proves affordable. Personally, I use it after training and periodically throughout the day. I have found that it improves my recovery. Also post-training I take a handful of branched-chain amino acids. They help the body repair itself as soon as possible. I also cycle my usage of creatine."* – Jamo Nezzar

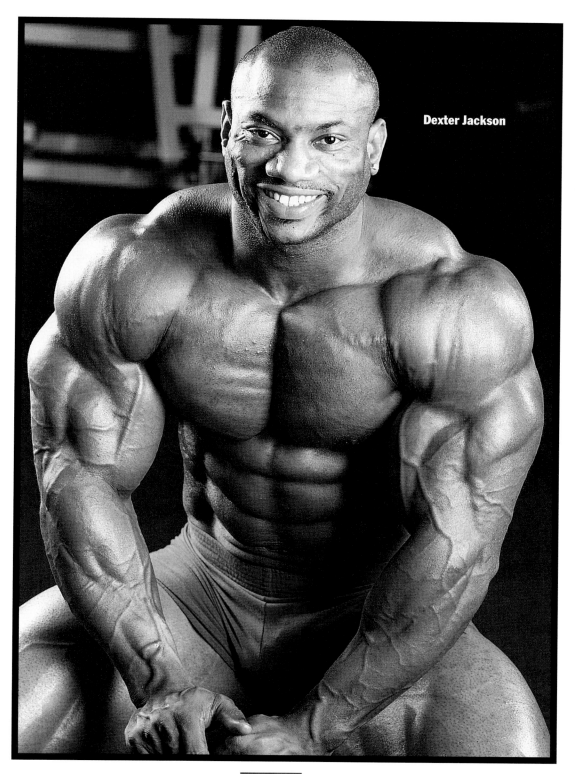

Dexter Jackson

5
MORE
MUSCLE MASS

One of the chief pursuits in body-building is to go *beyond average* and build more muscle. The general musclebuilding process exceeds normal to a great extent. However, even more muscle mass can be developed if you have the desire. To facilitate this goal, many bodybuilders embark upon a mass-building program. This is a specific training routine designed for a specific goal — to push the muscles from big to huge. Bodybuilders often work on adding muscle mass in the off-season, when they are not train- ing for an upcoming contest.

The pursuit of massive muscles is not unique to the sport of bodybuilding — football players and other power athletes seek to increase their mass for various reasons. But bodybuilding has the inside track on mass — and no one puts on as much dense muscle as a big bodybuilder. Height does not matter in this arena. Some

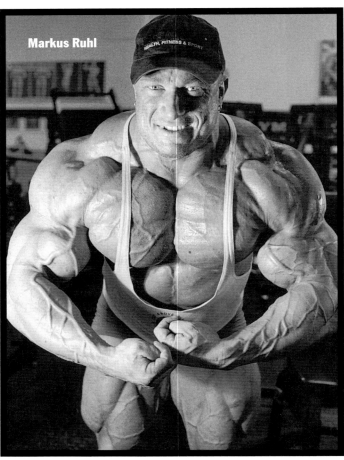

Markus Ruhl

bodybuilders who stand only 5'5" or 5'6" weigh more than 250 pounds. Now many six-footers weigh well over 300. Sure, lots of football players tip the scale at well over 300 pounds, but their stomach, hips and glutes carry most of the weight. Not so with bodybuilders.

Some 250-300+ pound bodybuilders still have good abs. That's lean mass!

Some bodybuilders have fairly lean hips and a moderate waistline — even at 250 to 325 pounds! Yes, some can even display a six-pack at 300 pounds. Bodybuilding size is muscle size. Getting massive does not simply mean getting bigger or weighing more. Mass in the bodybuilding realm translates to more muscle – a lot more muscle.

You can build your muscles up to a larger size than they are right now. Of course genetics plays a part, but everyone can realize tremendous gains from their current state.

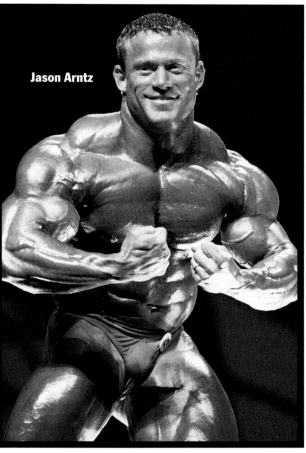

Jason Arntz

Mass Tracks

There are two basic tracks to building mass in the bodybuilding arena. One is to bulk up, gaining a good deal of size, and then cut off the excess bodyfat gained to reveal the lean muscles. The other track is to gradually and slowly add more muscle mass. There are proponents of both sides of the issue, and both will be discussed. The opinions of the professionals and what they have found to be effective will be featured in this chapter.

Early Mass

Another common approach to putting on body mass is to do so early in the game. The sooner you can attain a good deal of mass in your bodybuilding career, the better. The best time to specifically target the mass process is shortly after your first year or so of training. The initial entry into muscle-building should be focused on building a strong foundation, learning the various lifting techniques, the dietary approach, how to incorporate different workout schemes and various training tools, etc. Once you have gained some experience and your body has made the initial surge of growth, that is a good time to go for a second surge of growth – particularly in the area of mass. In fact this is the best time to make a move on upping your mass. However, if you have been lifting for quite some time and did not take advantage of this ideal time to gain mass, that does not mean you are forever doomed to a smaller body. You can still make substantial gains with a specific mass-building program. If you are a novice, however, seek to build that mass base early.

You can always add to the foundation you currently have built up and various mass-training cycles are popular. Professional bodybuilders strive to add another six to 12 pounds of muscle a year. For instance, Lee Priest noted in a *Max Sports Mag* interview that he was gaining seven to 12 pounds annually and

Most professional bodybuilders are toward the peak of their attainable size; a novice has a lot more room to grow.

happy with those gains. This type of progress is not accomplished during a precontest period – it comes in the off-season. The pros don't take all year to gain that weight, they do so in a short off-season cycle. If you are fairly new to training you can expect to make a lot more gains than that. The professionals are toward the peak of their attainable size. They are almost maxed out and still push it for even a few more strands of muscle gain. These massive monsters are very happy to be able to expand that mass by another 10 pounds or so. A novice trainer, on the other hand, is nowhere near the maximum attainable muscle mass and will likely make some significant gains.

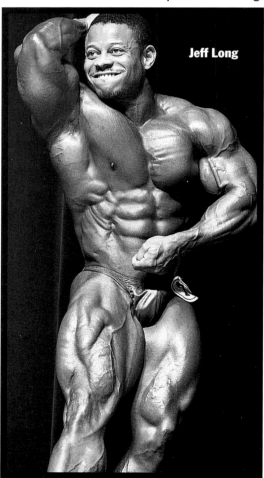

Jeff Long

Dorian Yates states he put on between 20 and 25 pounds of muscle in his first year of training, and says the average trainee should be able to put on 15 to 25 pounds, with a gain of 10 to 15 the following year. He notes that the amount of muscle gained each year will most likely decrease as the body adapts. If you add up Dorian's projection for the possibility of weight gain by a novice, it comes to 25 to 40 pounds of muscle in just a couple of years. That's a lot of muscle!

Don't make the common mistake of going after mass your first few sessions in the gym. The very idea of getting huge can be exciting, but go after the size in the proper training sequence. Give your body time to learn the mechanics of sound lifting. Give your body time to adjust to a new diet. Then make the move for mass. Before you get started on a specialized mass-building program, consider some insight from the really big guys.

Mass-Building Techniques of the Pros

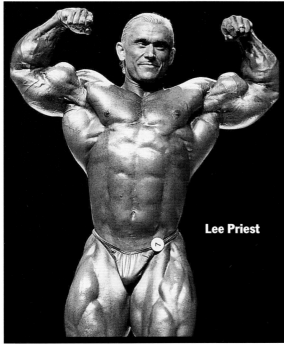

Lee Priest

Building muscle mass is an art. It takes both insight and intensity to turn the corner and gain that mass. Lee Priest stands roughly 5'4", and during the off-season weighs between 270 and 285 pounds. That's incredible. How does he do it? His ambition is "to do the best I can and to get progressively bigger." In a *Max Sports Mag* interview, Priest revealed his size training approach:

"I stick with the basic stuff, and in the off-season I train really heavy, bulk up big, and put on a lot of bodyfat. This last time I got up to 285 pounds and people said I'd never be able to train down and lose it, but when I've bulked up heavy I've always wound up with 10 pounds of muscle. You've really got to force-feed the muscles. Eating clean all year you'll be able to put on a couple of pounds of muscle … I'm concerned with my weight at only very specific times, and those are contest times. That's when it counts. Off-

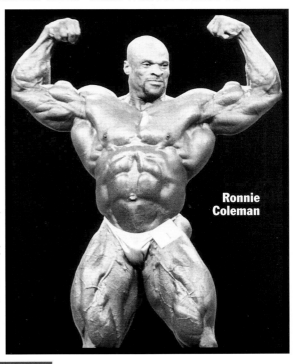

Ronnie Coleman

season I don't care how I look. They can call me a fat pig, which they do, but then comes contest time and they're all kissing my ass and saying how they knew I could get in shape. Whatever … You see Dorian and Nasser bulk up heavy and come out in superb shape, so it works."

Multi-Mr. Olympia Ronnie Coleman on Building Arm Mass

Ronnie Coleman pointed out in *Flex* magazine that the standard barbell curl is not his ideal tool for building massive biceps. "Cheating on barbell curls means that at certain times during the course of a rep the biceps are given an easy if not free ride. Based on the preceding thought, I came to the conclusion that cable work provided the required dual facilities of isolating the biceps while allowing them to remain under constant stress throughout the completion of each set. I start my routine with one-arm cable curls … My second exercise is bar cable curls. In terms of adding bulk throughout the entire biceps muscle, I find this movement to be superior (for reasons outlined previously) to the standard barbell curl."

Eating For Muscle Size From Jamo Nezzar

Jamo Nezzar has a fantastic physique — lean lines, yet massive muscle bellies. Here is his advice on eating for size.

Bulk-up diet for beginners:

(Use this diet if you are following the beginner training program.)

• First of all, eat for quality not quantity.

• Try to take in as much protein as you can.

• Eat about five meals spread throughout the day.

• Drink lots of water.

• Protein: You should eat 40 grams of protein per meal in the form of chicken (skinless), fish, eggs, and a good whey protein powder.

• Carbohydrates: rice, pasta, potatoes and oats.

• Fibrous carbs: should be in the form of fresh salad and vegetables.

• Fruit: bananas, apples and oranges.

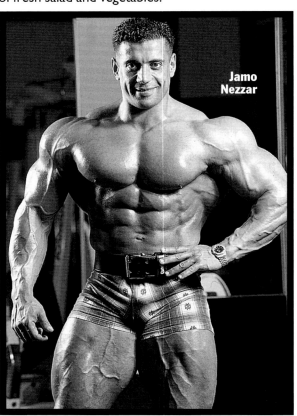

Jamo Nezzar

Meal 1: oats and skim milk, 4 eggs (1 yolk), 1 banana, coffee or tea

Meal 2: protein shake, 1 banana, 1/2 cup of dry oats

Meal 3: 2 chicken breasts (skinless), steamed rice, vegetables, large glass of water

Meal 4: protein shake, 1 banana, 1/2 cup of dry oats

Meal 5: fish or chicken salad, steamed vegetables, potatoes

Meal 6: 10 grams of glutamine, whey protein shake

Says Jamo on the importance of gutting it out to take it to the next level necessary to force the development of massive size, "At the Ironman this year I weighed 238 pounds. My next contest will once again be the Ironman. That gives me one whole year of training, eating and sleeping to get ready for that day. The plan is that I gain another 14 pounds by then. I expect to be over 250 onstage. At this level great genes are not enough. It goes without saying that to have gotten this far all the athletes must be gifted. From here on in it comes down to hard graft in the gym – day in and day out – remaining focused, staying injury free, and of course, determination."

How bad do you want to get big? Real bad? It takes a lot of willpower to pack on the amount of mass you want. It takes the use of *heavy metal.*

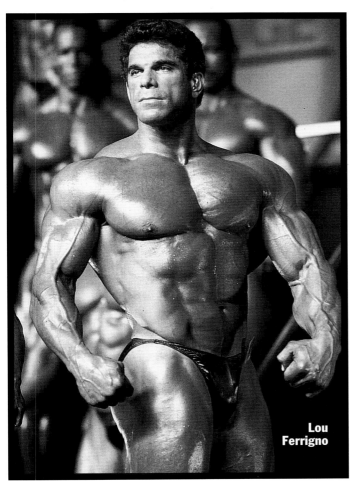

Lou Ferrigno

The Strength/Mass Connection
Lou Ferrigno, the only guy massive enough to play the role of the Incredible Hulk, knows a thing or two about massive size. He competed in the Olympia at a bodyweight of 318 pounds! Lou, one of the biggest in the bodybuilding world, notes, "At the most basic level, it is necessary to gain strength in order to gain mass. It's that simple. Get stronger and you'll get bigger. There's a direct correlation between the amount of weight you use in your exercises and the size of the muscles that lift it ... You'll need short and heavy workouts to gain weight: heavy to stimulate growth, short to allow recuperation as well as growth. The easiest way to do short workouts is to restrict them to basic exercises that work two or more large muscle groups at the same time."

Many bodybuilders utilize power-lifting movements during the mass training phase. Ronnie Coleman is noted for benching 405 pounds, squatting 585, and deadlifting 675 – for 10 reps each set! Greater strength will bring more muscle mass. The combination of the three power lifts in a bodybuilding routine can yield impressive results. Lou Ferrigno's suggested mass-building course includes the three (bench, squat and deadlift) along with bent-over rows, shrugs, barbell curls, military presses and calf-machine raises.

As Stuart McRobert points out, "To get bigger muscles, you need to build muscles that are much stronger – not just a few pounds stronger. That means a 25 percent increase in all your poundages if you want to see significant size increases and 50 percent if you want to see substantial growth. At the same time you must maintain impeccable form."

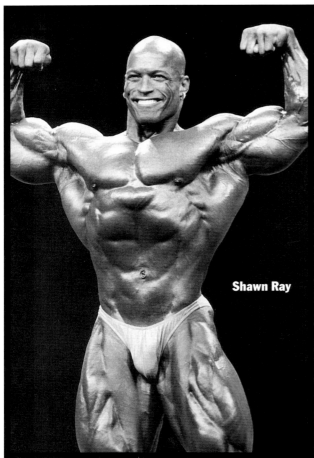

Shawn Ray

Chest-Training for Mass

Shawn Ray shares his advice on basic chest-training for mass at his Web site: "Three exercises, 4 sets, 8 reps. This is my golden rule of thumb when packing on mass! Keep it basic and simple. Pyramid the weight up to your max set. Begin by stretching the pecs out with some easy shoulder rotations and pectoral movements without weight resistance. When thoroughly warmed up, begin your first lift with a set of 15 reps to get the flow of blood into the chest. Basic lifts include bench, incline, flyes and dips. I like to use a mix of barbell and dumbells in my workouts for greater variation in working the muscle from different angles."

Many professionals point to the need for concentration and a strong attitude when pushing for mass. So does Shawn. "When training chest you must think big, strong and massive. See *yourself* pushing the weight through the range of motion to the finish position."

Off-Season Size

- Roland Kickinger weighs in at 320 in the off-season at a height of 6'4".
- Kevin Levrone weighs approximately 265 pounds at 5'9".
- Jay Cutler weighs roughly 275 in the off-season at 5'9".
- Ronnie Coleman goes close to 300 in the off-season at a height of 5'11".
- Jean-Pierre Fux has a similar weight of 300 pounds in the off-season, also at a height of 5'11".
- Jimmy Mentis is roughly 305 in the off-season at 6'1" in height.
- Flex Wheeler at 5' 9" is close to 250 pounds in the off-season.
- Craig Titus is also 5'9" but close to 270 pounds in the off-season.
- Nasser El Sonbaty weighs around 325 in the off-season at 5'11".
- Ernie Taylor weighs around 285 pounds in the off-season and is 5'8."
- Lee Priest weighs around 285 in the off-season at 5'4".
- Gunter Schlierkamp goes approximately 300 off-season at 6'1".

If you ran a rough composite of this group, the average off-season size would be around 285 pounds. Compare that to the off-season size of the early Mr. Olympias like Larry Scott, who didn't push much past the 200-pound barrier. A few years later Arnold and Sergio were thought to be monsters in the off-season at 235 to 250 pounds. These days a bodybuilder with Arnold's height of 6'2" would be thought of as quite small at 240 pounds – today's 5'11" to 6'1" gang weigh 300 to 320 pounds during the off-season.

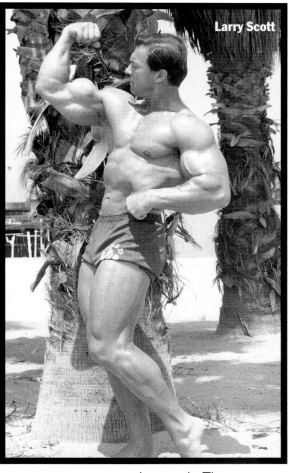

Larry Scott

Repetition Range

In general, a lower repetition range is suggested by most professionals when pursuing mass. Skip La Cour prefers a range of 4 to 6 reps. The one exception is the high-repetition squat, where 20 reps are used to stimulate the metabolism (as well as the body's biggest muscle group, the thighs). The 20-repetition squat has been used by hundreds of bodybuilders to prompt new muscle growth. There are even books touting the benefits of high-repetition squatting.

In general, particularly for the upper body, a lower repetition range is called for. Do either 5 to 7 repetitions, such as the range Brian Buchannan and Lee Haney have found productive for size gains, or 4 to 6 reps as La Cour prefers. Shawn Ray suggests 8 repetitions for massing up the chest. The upper end of the rep range for mass-building in the upper body should be no more than 8 reps, and generally less. The lower rep range is a mix of the power and strength-producing effects of lower reps with the low end of the size-producing range. In general, higher repetitions will help definition, endurance and other factors, but not work as well for size. Again, the one exception is the high-repetition squat sets and the occasional (brief) high-rep shock cycle.

For sparking growth, lower the repetition range and increase the poundage.

Number of Sets

The number of sets done should also be less when mass is the goal. You are not trying to win a marathon – you are trying to build muscle. According to Dorian Yates, "Most people are overtraining in sets and reps and undertraining in intensity. They're training too long and too often. Whatever you're currently doing, cut the volume in half and raise your intensity level by 50 percent." Fewer sets can mean as low as 1 or 2 sets on some exercises, 3 to 4 on others. Do not make the novice mistake of increasing sets as you chase mass – decease the number of sets; Just make sure the ones you do get in are carried out with good form and all-out white-hot intensity.

Frequency

While the workload for building mass should be higher than average, the frequency should be less. Stuart McRobert points out that, if you hope to make gains, "you need more off days than on days." When training for mass, rest becomes even more important than usual. McRobert summarizes: "To get stronger muscles, you must train hard and briefly on the minimum of exercises so that you don't exceed your recovery ability. You must keep adding a tad of iron every week or two, year after year … as long as you want to build bigger

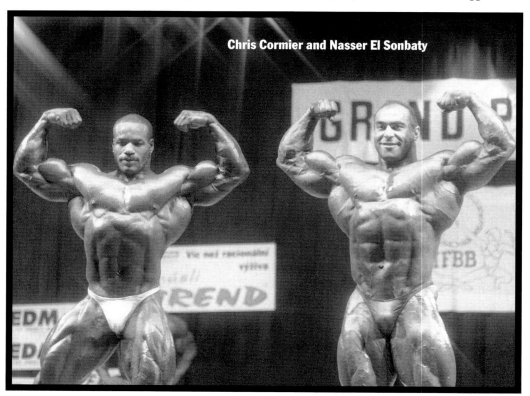

Chris Cormier and Nasser El Sonbaty

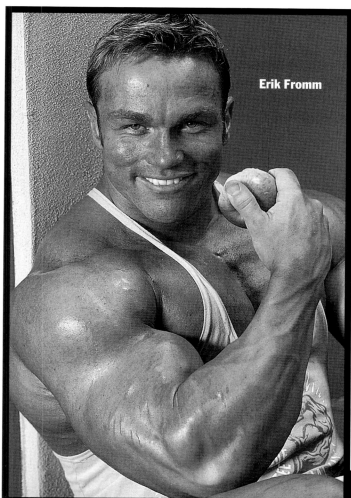
Erik Fromm

muscles. To be able to do that, however, you must be able to recover from your training. If you return to the gym before you've fully recovered, how can you add iron to the bar? If you can't add iron to the bar, how are you going to build the extra strength that yields bigger muscles?"

Time off, rest time, is an important factor in musclebuilding. It is twice as important in a mass-building cycle, so factor in at least one more day of rest between workouts than for a regular routine.

Focus

The focus of mass training needs to be centered on the major muscle groups. Target the naturally large muscles of the body – the back, the chest, and the thighs. Work briefly on the other muscle groups, but make the main thrust of your training attack on the big ones. By concentrating your training on these areas you will make the body respond in a big way.

Food

Bodybuilders agree almost universally that, in order to make a mass program successful, you will need to crank up the calories. Look at the intake of a top champion in contest training compared to the off-season – the calories are double – or even triple – for off-season training. Some trainers contend you will never get massive unless you increase your nutrient intake. The carbs need to be high to fuel the heavy-duty workouts as well as assist in recovery from the same workouts. Protein intake also needs to be high for the desired increase in muscle size, and fat content should be high. Take advantage of an extra protein drink or two during the day to keep the calories coming.

Take note: Although mass-training diets are high in calories from all three nutrient sources (fats, carbs, protein), this does not mean you have a license to eat anything. The goal is bigger muscles, not a bigger spare tire. Keep the increase in calories clean – from nutrient-dense sources. No junk food. Clean calories build muscles; junk food tears them down.

Jay Cutler reveals, "Even in the off-season I eat the same foods day in and day out. That's part of my discipline as a bodybuilder. I've learned what foods work best for me and I stay with them. During the off-season I eat a lot of egg whites and chicken breasts because those proteins work well with my body."

• For building mass, increase the poundage and lower the repetition range. Squats are the one exception – 20-rep squats can yield mass.
• Decrease the number of sets in a workout, but increase the intensity.
• Increase the amount of time between workouts and dedicate your days off to rest and recuperation.
• Increase caloric intake but maintain a habit of eating clean, nutritious foods. Stay away from junk food.
• Focus the mass-training routine on the bigger muscle groups such as back, legs and chest.

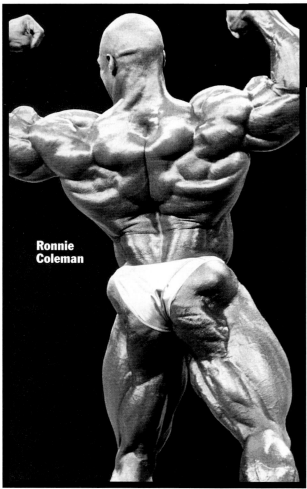

Ronnie Coleman

Thoughts From the Pros on Building Mass

On the basics: *"I can't help how I look in the off-season. I train heavy and stick to the basic work – which is hard basic work. Some people get lazy. When I first came over here I was dazzled by all the machines. I began to ignore the basics and figured that the machines would work just as well, but I could see that the results were not the same. Then I had to go back to basic free-weight movements like barbell rows, curls, squats, dumbell presses, etc. It seems everybody these days would rather use a leg-press machine than do squats, or an arm-curl machine than do heavy barbell curls."* – Lee Priest in *Confessions of a Priest*, *maxsportsmag.com*

On biceps mass: *"A beginner's need for sheer size is more urgent than building hardness and density. The lower rep range and heavier poundages will fulfill that need."* – Ronnie Coleman

On basics for growth: *"As I said, the days back in Algeria did serve their purpose. They taught me a lot about the basics of training. Because the gyms were not equipped with the latest machines, we had to make do with all the old-fashioned compound moves. Actually, to say we made do is not fair. You will find that most of the top guys are still using those moves to this day. I know I still am."* – Jamo Nezzar

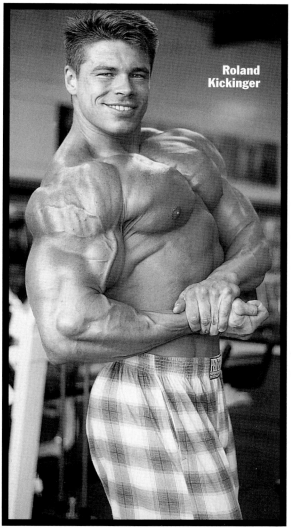

Roland Kickinger

The mass equation: *"Gaining muscular mass and strength requires a combination of four very important factors: proper training, proper nutrition, sufficient recuperation time, and the correct mental attitude."* – Lou Ferrigno

Nutrition is vital for mass: *"Bodybuilding and weight training involves more than just gym work. You'd better be prepared to provide your muscles with the nutrition they need for growth."* – Jimmy Mentis

Six square: *"I must eat six times a day."* – Roland Kickinger

Journal: *"To become a massively developed bodybuilder takes time – a number of years in most cases. I do believe, however, that the amount of time it would take any person to develop his fullest potential would be reduced dramatically if he were to keep a training journal from the very first day he started."* –The late Mike Mentzer

Heavy training for natural bodybuilders: *"Getting progressively stronger is the only way a natural bodybuilder will gain mass. I train as heavy as possible and take every set to failure."* – Skip La Cour

Realistic goal: *"A realistic goal for mass-building is to pack on one-half to one pound of bodyweight per week during your growth cycle. If you are gaining more weight than that, you are eating too much food – and your gains will be mostly fat."* – Chris Aceto

6

THE NEXT LEVEL –
ADVANCED TRAINING TECHNIQUES

Musclebuilding is quite a unique endeavor in that you must consistently change your approach. Yeah, it can be a bummer; just when you think you have learned the program, you realize it's time to change. Unlike many sports in which you learn to master the moves and then simply work on doing them again and again, in bodybuilding the maneuvers are subject to change. *When?* Just about the time you have worked through the basic training phase, and a good mass-building phase, it will be time to try some-

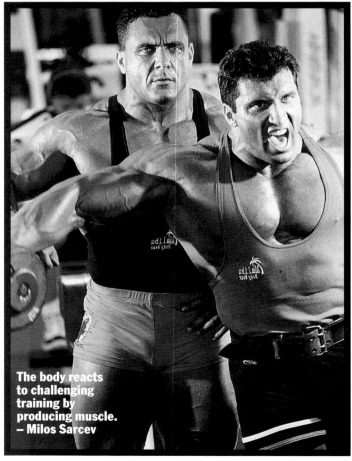

The body reacts to challenging training by producing muscle. – Milos Sarcev

thing new. *Why?* Because the body does not allow continuous muscle growth. In fact the body won't produce muscle growth at all unless it is given a pretty good reason. Once it has adapted and adjusted to the basic training, it quits growing and you have to push hard just to break even. A mass phase will bring about more growth, but even that will roll to a stop after a period of time. The body reacts to challenging workouts by producing muscle to handle the workload of training – then it figures out how much muscle is necessary, and won't give any more than that.

Milos Sarcev points out, "Muscles are highly adaptive; they quickly become immune to routine stresses." Many people quit here because moving ahead at this junction is difficult. However, it can be done if you apply certain advanced training techniques.

Muscle Confusion

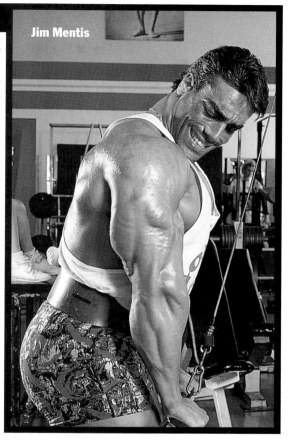

Jim Mentis

One of the main principles you can use to advance muscle growth once you graduate beyond basic training is *muscle confusion.* Jimmy Mentis points out why he uses this technique: "I like to use different exercises once in a while, so I do not get stuck in a certain routine. I use a Weider principle called confusion training. This is where you do different exercises or change the order of your exercises all the time. That keeps the muscles on their toes and they will respond better."

Most professionals use the muscle confusion technique in some form or another. In fact muscle confusion lies at the heart of most advanced training technique variations.

"Muscles are highly adaptive; they quickly become immune to routine stresses." – Milos Sarcev

The key to confusing the muscles is to take them out of the ordinary routine. You control a number of variables that will allow you to do just that. For example, Shawn Ray suggests changing the repetition and weight scheme, exercise order, or even using different exercises every workout. Muscle confusion is basic in premise – give the muscles a challenge they have not faced before. The body becomes familiar with workout patterns fairly quickly; your main concern is to keep the muscles stimulated workout after workout.

Microblast the Muscles

The longer you have been lifting weights, the more stimulation your muscles need to spark new strength and size. If you get stuck at a certain level of training volume, guess what? Your body will also be stuck. You cannot expect good results if your training volume stays the same. Unfortunately a very real paradox exists – although you need more volume to boost the body to new muscle size, you also need more rest. Don't continue to hammer away at your physique workout after workout – that's not the answer when your gains have come to a stop. In fact that approach will make the gains stop even sooner and you'll be stuck at the plateau even longer.

The answer is *not* to cut the volume – remember, less training volume equals less muscular development. The answer here lies is *microblast training*, which is actually an increase in intensity. You crank up the workload on your muscles more than ever – add weight to the bar, another set, deeper concentration, and perhaps a high-repetition set to top it all off. But unlike the normal routine, you don't work that muscle group for several days, taking as many as six to 12 days off before working it again. You blast them out of orbit, then get 'em a lot of rest. This technique is great. You get into a workout/rest routine that fosters new muscle gains.

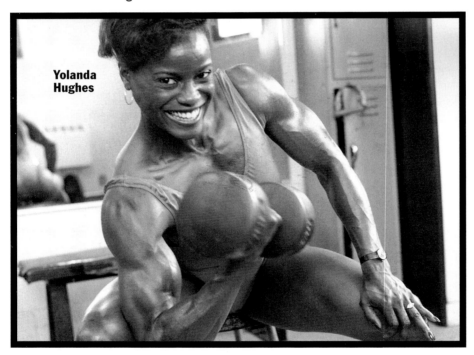

Yolanda
Hughes

Priority Training

Priority training involves putting a priority on weak areas of your physique. No one is perfect and every bodybuilder has a chink in his or her armor somewhere, an area that could use more work. Priority training involves going into "maintenance mode" with other muscle groups while you focus most of the training time and energy on your weak spots. Most novices get stuck pumping out set after set for the fun of it – for muscles like biceps and chest – and tend to overlook their weak areas. This tends to exacerbate the problem. The body gets totally out of control, lacking any real symmetry. To overcome this situation, try priority training. You will need strong commitment to bypass your favorite exercises and zero in on bodyparts that need improvement. If you want to compete, this discipline is an absolute necessity. In fact an off-kilter physique detracts from the impressive areas. Champion bodybuilder Chris Cormier states, "I strive to build all my bodyparts symmetrically and in proportion to each other." For that type of result you will need to prioritize your training.

Priority training, when a weak muscle group is trained with first priority. Is the perfect solution for muscle imbalances in either strength or size. Flex Wheeler incorporated priority training in his bid to add even more mass to his incredible physique, and succeeded in netting 17 pounds of pure muscle. How is priority training accomplished? You can go about priority training in several ways. Justin Leonard points out one approach:

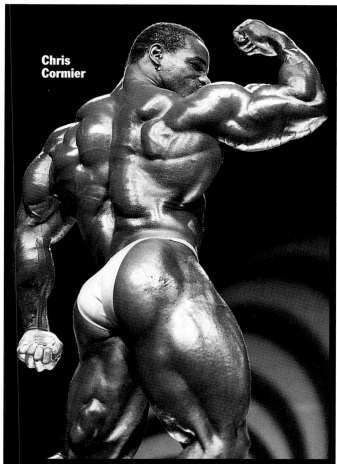

Chris Cormier

"One example of priority training is to train the weakest bodypart at the beginning of a workout week. For example, most people begin their week with a chest routine on Monday. Some trainers have skinny leg muscles which do not match their well-sized upper body. If they trained legs [as opposed to chest] early in the week, when energy and motivation levels are high, they could expect better results.

"Another way to prioritize is to train or focus on one particular bodypart more than others. It's an easy fix. If you know your legs are lacking, do the same thing you did to get your chest to look the way it does. You may need to train legs twice a week or spend more time per workout training them."

One more thought on the use of priority training – the bodypart first up in the training rotation gets the best blood, which equals the best pump.

"I strive to build all my bodyparts symmetrically and in proportion to each other." – Chris Cormier

The Pump

If you have been training for any length of time, you will notice that during your workouts your muscles expand and get bigger. This phenomenon is what the professionals aim for in their training sessions. The more advanced you are, the better pump you can attain in your muscles. Flex Wheeler says, if I can achieve a great pump with 30-pound dumbells, then that's what I'll use. Specific training for the pump brings about impressive results. The pump comes from concentrated volume. As noted earlier in this book, when exercising, waste products and lactic acid are produced in the muscle cells. This accumulation is commonly referred to as the pump, and the situation eventually leads to muscle failure. Meanwhile blood is rushing to the area being worked. Blood flow is key to a great pump and is vital. Ron Brown points out the progress of the pump:

"Regardless of how intensely you think you are training, there is one sign that will never fail to tell you if you are training intensely enough – increased blood flow into the muscle, physiologically called hyperemia, a.k.a. *The pump!* The pump is not just a side effect of exercise. For musclebuilding purposes the pump is the main goal of exercise. No one can say for sure why pumping up an undeveloped muscle will make it grow, but experience shows that it does ... every time, always, no exceptions! (All other elements like proper food and rest being equal, of course.)

"By the way, testosterone is not necessary for this type of muscle growth to occur. Testosterone is a hormone that creates new muscle fibers in boys as they develop into adults. These new fibers are made out of permanent structural proteins. Testosterone has little effect in creating new fibers in adults. The type of growth we are talking about here is the increased size of existing fibers in both men and women, not the creation of new muscle fibers. This enlargement of existing fibers is due to the addition of labile or temporary proteins (mainly actomyosin). The pump is the best way to deliver these proteins and other nutrients to the muscle fibers.

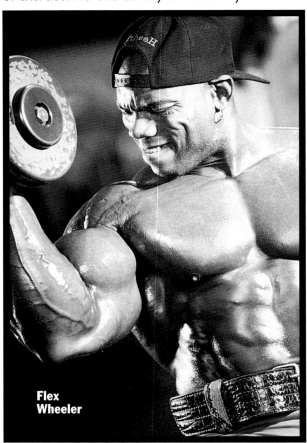

Flex
Wheeler

Achieving a pump requires strict attention to timing. Filling up your muscles with extra blood is like filling up a bucket with a hole in the bottom. Fluid has to flow into the vessel at a faster rate than what leaks out. That means you can't take a break and start socializing in the middle of working toward a pump. Work with maximum intensity until you achieve a pump. Then, when you can't get it pumped any more, quit exercising that muscle. Nothing deflates a pump quicker than overexercising."

The pump is king for advancing the muscle growth once you get beyond the basic and mass phases. Arnold Schwarzenegger accredited the pump as being the key to success in building mighty muscles.

Here's another way to look at it. The quicker you can obtain the pump, the better. Larry Scott stated that he aimed for the quickest pump in the shortest length of time.

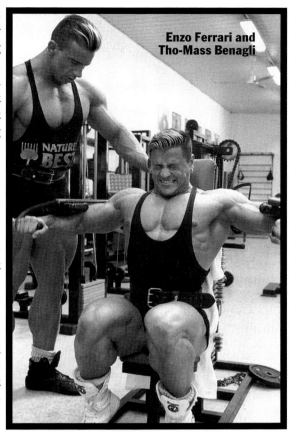

Enzo Ferrari and Tho-Mass Benagli

Drop Sets

One way to ensure your muscles get not only a pump but also a real blowout is to use drop sets. Drop sets also go by the name *strip sets* since weights are stripped off the bar (dumbells can also be used in descending poundages). Dramo13's online site provides a good how-to description: Strip sets should be done on the last or second last set of a bodypart and only about once a week, or once every second workout, ideally with a partner to help strip the plates off. Start with a heavy weight with which you can get 4 to 6 reps, and do as many as you can. Then strip about 10 percent of the weight off the bar and do as many reps as you can with that weight. Strip 10 to 20 percent off and rep out again. Take about three minutes' rest and do it all again.

Drop sets are used by many of the top professionals at various times in their training routines. You can drop the weight at a number of stages – the muscles burn up at about the third drop. Dr. Mauro Di Pasquale points to the use of the triple-drops as the best way to put on muscle mass. He describes one manner in which to employ this technique: "The drop set starts with a weight you can handle for just 5 reps and not 6. Then some weight is taken off and another 5 reps are done. Still more weight is removed and a final 5 reps are done. I usually stay on a triple-drop routine for six to ten weeks. Once the strength gains stop or I start getting too sore, I go on an eccentric-type training regimen."

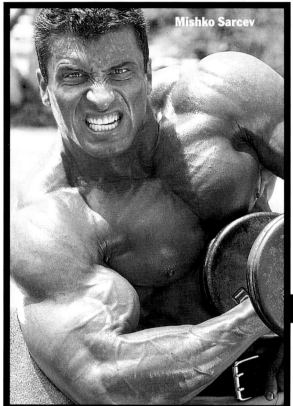

Mishko Sarcev

Dorian Yates would employ the triple drop in his hardcore workouts.

A similar training technique is called the down-the-rack approach, where progressively lighter dumbells are used in nonstop action until the muscles give out. They are a favorite tool of Ollie McClay in biceps work.

One key point in making drop sets and down-the-rack training successful is to maintain good form in each drop. By the second drop or so you will be in a lot of pain. You may be tempted to start letting momentum help you move the weight. Don't – make the muscles continue to do the work.

Slow Motion

A good way to introduce a new stimulus to your training is to simply slow down the speed at which you move through your reps. Some studies have indicated that slow-motion lifting does improve muscle strength due to the minimized momentum and maximized muscle tension. Slow-motion action forces the muscles into a new challenge, and therefore new growth. This type of training should not be done all the time (moderate speed is the best base) but can act as a great change of pace and produce good results for you. Mishko Sarcev reveals the following:

"You can vary the rep speed as you wish, but I've found it best to take a slow-motion approach: three or four seconds going up and three or four on the return … Your focus will remain on the working muscle."

"I've found it best to take a slow-motion approach; three or four seconds going up and three or four on the return."
– Mishko Sarcev

Pre-Exhaust Training

I initially came up with the pre-exhaust system as an advanced training technique. Here's how Wayne L. Westcott, PhD, discussed pre-exhaust and other forms of high-intensity training compared to standard training in his article on high-intensity training:

"Pre-exhaustion training is also designed to fatigue more muscle fibers than standard training. With this high-intensity technique you complete two successive exercise sets for the same muscle group. The first set is typically done with a rotary exercise that fatigues the target muscle group. The second set is conducted with a linear exercise that involves both the fatigued target muscle group and a fresh muscle group. For example, you may do a set of chest flyes to pre-exhaust the pectoralis major muscles. At the point of failure, you may immediately do a set of chest presses using both the fatigued pectoralis major muscles and the fresh triceps muscles. By incorporating different movement patterns and fresh muscles, pre-exhaustion produces greater fatigue in the target muscle group. Other effective pre-exhaust combinations include lateral raises followed by overhead presses for the deltoid muscles, pullovers followed by pulldowns for the latissimus dorsi, arm curls then chinups for biceps, arm extensions with dips for the triceps, and leg extensions followed by leg presses for the quadriceps. Conclusion: Our study with adults and seniors demonstrated significantly more strength development with breakdown training than with standard training. Although not researched, experience indicates that

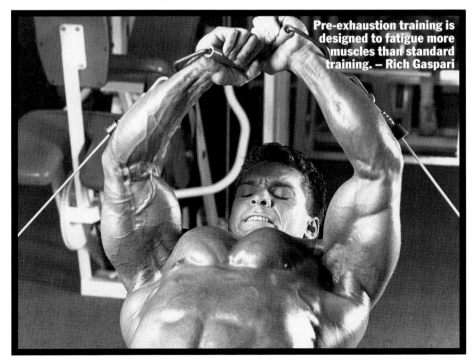

Pre-exhaustion training is designed to fatigue more muscles than standard training. – Rich Gaspari

assisted training and the pre-exhaust technique are also effective means of producing more muscle fiber involvement and promoting greater strength gains.

"In addition to the physiological adaptations associated with high-intensity strength exercise, there would appear to be psychological changes as well. That is, people who practice high-intensity techniques are likely to train harder than those who have not exercised in this manner. Because of the greater effort required by high-intensity strength exercise, it should not be overdone. A single breakdown set, a few assisted repetitions, and an occasional pre-exhaustion workout will be sufficient. Most important, be sure to do every repetition in standard and high-intensity exercises with proper technique and controlled movement speed."

Pre-exhaust training is a great way to break out of a rut or go beyond a sticking point. You can cycle this system into your training at various times throughout the year and expect good results.

Shock Training

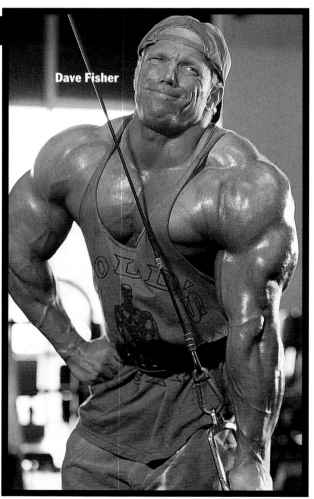

Dave Fisher

All training should be a type of shock to the body to some extent. However, there is a specific type of training where the body gets blasted out of the ball park. Shock training involves increasing either the number of exercises for a single muscle group, the repetition range, number of sets, or all three. This strategy is usually aimed at one muscle group at a time. For instance, a regular back-training session may involve 3 sets each of three different exercises. A shock routine could employ five exercises, 5 to 7 sets each.

Another approach is to choose a muscle group and do a set an hour throughout the whole day to overload that muscle with sudden stimulation. The late Vince Gironda noted that the arms, for instance, could grow noticeably on such a shock routine (provided abundant rest was incorporated afterward).

Shock training is totally intense. This technique should be employed on an infrequent basis only – with lots of time for rest and recuperation. Allow at least a week's rest for that muscle group after a shock-training session.

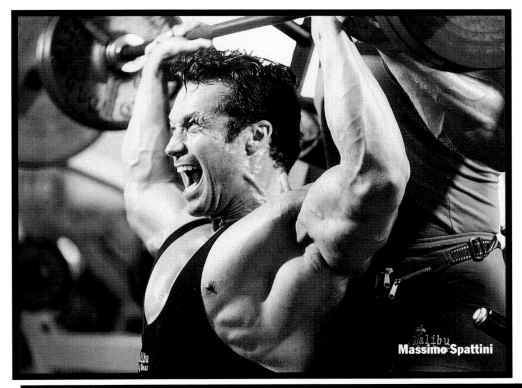

Massimo Spattini

Forced Reps

What do you do when you've taken the weights as far as you think you can humanly go? …You push it further with forced reps. Of course you need a training partner for this technique (don't try it alone). When you reach the point where you've gotten the last rep you can possibly manage, your partner will move in and help you get 2 to 4 more. This requires a savvy partner who knows how little pressure to take off the bar so you are still working hard. One strategy is to have your spotter assist you at the sticking points only, so you must do the rest of the work yourself throughout the full range of motion. This is one of the most intense types of training around – enjoy!

Negative Reps

A negative approach can build positive growth. The negative half of a rep is also called the eccentric portion. Here you focus on the lowering of the weight, the downstroke of the lifting movement. The idea is, you can handle much more weight in lowering it than you can in raising it, and the task of handling heavy weights both strengthens the muscle and prepares it for heavier weights in the future. As with forced reps, a partner is necessary for best results. Negative reps should be used in cycles, not as the main base of a training program.

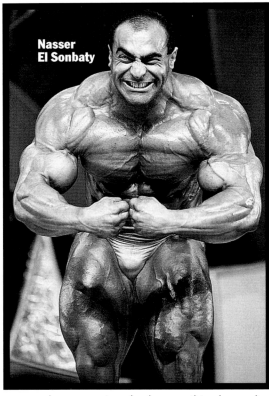

Nasser
El Sonbaty

Partial Reps

Most exercises should be carried out through the full range of motion. The muscles should bear the brunt of the work throughout the arc of the lift, and back down to the bottom of the repetition. However, partial reps do have a place in weight training. Most professionals incorporate partials at one time or another. Dorian was a big fan. Aaron Maddron uses them at the end of a set to failure. Partial reps employ only a portion of the arc of the lift. That can be any part of the range – midpoint, beginning or end phase of the repetition. Partial reps allow you to take the muscles a little further than if you just quit when you can't do any more full repetitions. Partial reps can also help build up the pump more completely, and give the muscle being worked a super deep burn. Some bodybuilders keep moving the bar until it almost has to be pried out of their hands! Partials are generally done at the end of a workout (although used for the first two stages of 21s before going to full repetitions). Experiment with partial movements and see what type of response your muscles have.

Peak Contraction

Can you say, *squeeeeeze?* The squeeze is the action of peak contraction – squeezing the muscle at the most intense phase of the repetition. Once the muscle is tight, you give it an extra squeeze and hold it for a painful second or two. Contracting the muscle as hard as you can is painful, but stimulates more muscle growth. Of course it would be difficult to do an entire workout in this manner. Nasser El Sonbaty makes it a point to put the peak contraction repetitions after the power and mass movements. For super pain, hit a few peak contractions, then follow through nonstop with full range of motion reps after that.

To sum it all up, employ a variety of advanced techniques and tricks to stimulate the muscle and you can expect new growth. One of the quickest ways to get past a training plateau is to bring in an advanced technique for forcing new muscle growth. Do not consider experimenting until you have gotten beyond basic training and the mass-gaining stages.

• Muscles initially grow to a certain point, then the gains taper off.
• You must build a solid base of muscle before moving up to advanced techniques.
• The best way to jump-start your muscles to new growth is to employ advanced techniques.
• The basis for starting new gains lies in muscle confusion — getting out of the same old routine rut.
• Learn the principles behind advanced techniques first, then incorporate them into your workout.

Thoughts From the Pros on Advanced Training

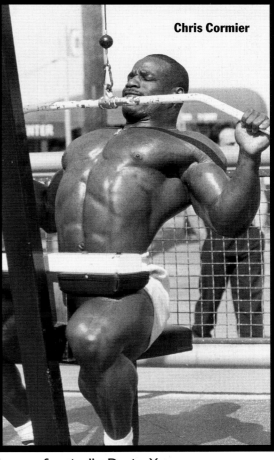

Chris Cormier

On quality training: *"Before I was some sort of a serious bodybuilding competitor I would just train for mass. As the years went by I also had to start looking at shape and quality of the muscle."* – Jimmy Mentis

On change: *"When you first start training you make phenomenal gains ... Eventually, however, your body adapts to the level of training stress you are exposing it to; your progress begins to slow and perhaps even stop ... Once you hit a plateau you will make no progress unless you change your approach."* – Shawn Ray

More on change: *"I'm never dogmatic when it comes to my training routine. If I discover something new, I don't hesitate to use it."* – Flex Wheeler

Range of motion: *"My emphasis is less on lifting the weight and more on achieving a full range of motion."* – Dorian Yates

On variety: *"If you use enough variety, plateauing may become a nonissue."* – Mishko Sarcev

Various strategies: *"I attribute my success to doing consistent heavy work for over 16 years. I've been lifting since I was 12 years old, and I've always paid close attention to different training strategies."* – Chris Cormier

7

THE REST OF
THE PACKAGE

Bodybuilding consists of a lot more than simply working out and eating right. There are several ancillary elements that also play a role in the overall package of a fully developed physique. Incorporating these other elements into your musclebuilding approach will make it much more complete. As always, many have already "been there and done that" and you can learn from their knowledge. While these additional aspects of bodybuilding are not in the spotlight as much as the star elements – weightlifting and eating nutritiously – they can add up to give you that extra edge to make your physique look even better. Consider incorporating some or all of them into your physique package to maximize your routine.

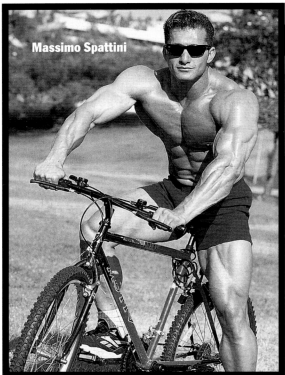

Massimo Spattini

Aerobic Activity

Aerobics is a tool many bodybuilders use to burn off unwanted bodyfat and assist the process of making the body leaner. When some people hear the term *aerobics* they think of television fitness cheerleaders dancing around in tights. In reality aerobics is a broad category. As fitness expert Covert Bailey points out, "In practical terms any exercise is aerobic if it 1) lasts at least 12 minutes without stopping, 2) gets you breathing deeply but not out of breath, and 3) uses the muscles of the thighs and buttocks." Bailey also notes the aerobic zone runs from 65 to 80 percent of maximum heart beat range.

One of the key uses of aerobic training is to burn bodyfat, the other is for overall physical health. In general, weight training does not use fat as fuel. After the workout there is a nice burn of bodyfat due to postworkout recovery, but during the workout the fuel source for moving the weights is glycogen, not fat. With aerobics the opposite is true. Fat is used as the primary fuel source, particularly the longer the session lasts. That is, in the beginning of any aerobic-style activity the fuel source is mainly converted carbs (ATP, glycogen). However, the body switches fuel tanks at about the 12 to 20 minute

"I'm a firm believer in getting up early and going for a fast walk, bike ride or jog to get the blood flowing and bump up the metabolism. Maintain a consistent weight-training schedule, but alternate your exercises so your body doesn't get used to any one routine." – Carol Ann Weber

mark, and from 20 to 30 minutes on out, fat is the fuel of choice for the body and glycogen use drops off. For burning off bodyfat during a workout, aerobic-style training is great.

Most bodybuilders do some aerobic work during regular training, with more aerobics added as a competition draws near, and little to none in the off-season/mass-building phase. However, some bodybuilders do no aerobic activities at all. One bodybuilding writer Greg Merritt states, "Excessive aerobics can rob you of muscle-growing rest and mass-building calories. As a result, it's usually best to avoid running, bike riding and other concentrated aerobics when trying to gain mass … Never do aerobics on the same day that you train thighs."

Light aerobic work, on the other hand, greatly enhances fat-burning. You'll often see a bodybuilder on a stationary bike, particularly as contest time approaches. Another tool is powerwalking (walking at a fast pace), which is ideal for burning off bodyfat without pushing the body too far. Some of the hardcore aerobic exercises can rob the muscles; lighter aerobic activities such as power-walking and stationary biking do not, and are a great manner in which to get rid of that last bit of bodyfat. Shawn Ray recommends cardio/aerobic work four times a week for no less than 20 minutes per session. Dorian Yates used aerobic workouts, even in the off-season. Make aerobics part of your weekly training package.

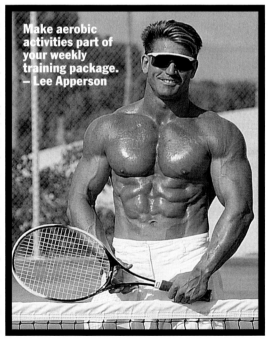

Make aerobic activities part of your weekly training package. – Lee Apperson

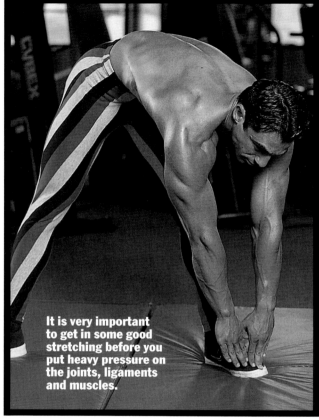

It is very important to get in some good stretching before you put heavy pressure on the joints, ligaments and muscles.

Stretching

Stretching is an important pre-exercise action taken to get the muscles prepared for the workout. Lou Ferrigno notes that stretching before a workout sends a signal to the muscles that they are about to receive stimulation. He raises the body temperature, which helps prevent injury. Never underestimate the importance of a good stretching session before you put heavy pressure on the joints, ligaments and muscles. Very few bodybuilders start a workout without first stretching for at least a few minutes.

However, stretching has gained status as a manner in which to help the muscles grow even more. The stereotypical muscle-bound bodybuilder has been pervasive, but in actuality many bodybuilders are quite flexible. Who can forget Tom Platz touching his head to his shins? The more flexible you are, the better. Stretching is now recognized as a complementary training tool. Many bodybuilders have actually incorporated stretching into the workout itself. Several say they believe stretching is responsible for adding a bit more size to their muscles. Stretching takes only a couple of extra minutes, but brings about many benefits.

Tanning

A solid tan looks great — no two ways about it. More important for the competitive bodybuilder, a solid tan makes the muscles stand out against the glare of the posing lights. A good tan enhances the appearance of the muscles. Compare two bodies that have the exact same muscle build, but one is a pasty white and the other has a nice even tan. The tanned physique looks far better. A skin tone that is too pale conveys a sense of illness; a tan conveys the idea of outdoor activity and health. But hold on a minute — the pale-skinned person may actually be healthier! Although a tan is needed, due to the problem of skin cancer, you don't want to forfeit your life over a darker shade of brown. Too much time in the sun or in a tanning bed can harm the body, exposing it to dangerous skin cancers like melanoma. One alternative chosen by many bodybuilders is to get a certain base tan, then use a "tan in a bottle" to add another layer of bronze. If you choose to enter a contest you will have to come in with a good dark color. Carefully combine some tanning with the bottled version of tanning for the effect that gives you both color and some degree of skin safety.

Posing

Any sculptor who has a creation worth looking at wants to show it off. The same is true in bodybuilding, where the sculpture created is the body. Posing is the form in which the body's muscles are exhibited. In order to compare the top physiques, an event has evolved where the muscles are displayed in various configurations in order to show that the physique has been fully developed. A team of judges rate the physiques in comparison, score each entrant's physique during a series of posing rounds, and then decide on the winner in the final round. *Eastcoastmuscle.com* notes, "There are three posing rounds required in prejudging (or preliminary judging) in bodybuilding competitions: 1) the symmetry or relaxed round, 2) the mandatory or compulsory round, and 3) the individual posing routine.

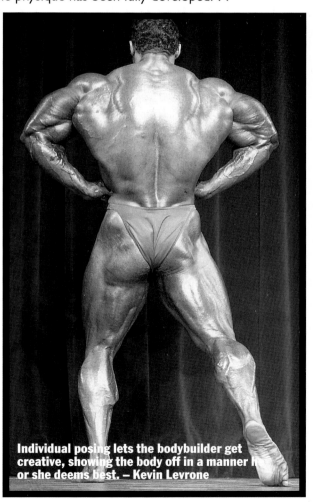

Individual posing lets the bodybuilder get creative, showing the body off in a manner he or she deems best. – Kevin Levrone

The first two rounds carry the most influence in judging. Posing involves flexing the muscles to maximum size, or shrinking the muscles down as in the area of the midsection, as well as presenting the body in a semi-relaxed condition. In the mandatory round everyone has to go through the same poses in order to let the various physiques be measured against the others. Individual posing lets the bodybuilder get creative, showing the body off in a manner he or she deems best. Music plays a big part in creating the mood in the individual posing round.

Finally there is the posedown, where the finalists vie for the judges' attention. The pushing and jostling for position in this round almost reminds you of a real battle. At last the winners are announced in ascending order. Competitions usually feature winners of different weight classes (in the early days of bodybuilding the group was divided by height), and then they announce one overall winner.

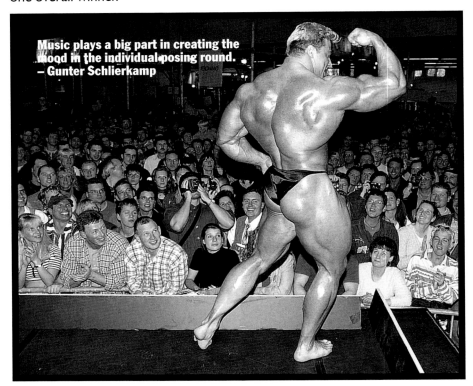

Music plays a big part in creating the mood in the individual posing round.
— Gunter Schlierkamp

No more than 5 percent of all bodybuilders compete, but posing is not just for them. Posing in itself is tough work and a great way to cap off a hard workout. It helps maintain the pump and lets you see your progress. Many gyms feature walls of mirrors — not only to let the trainees follow their form, but also to allow opportunity for posing and checking out the muscles. If you feel a bit shy initially, pose at home. When your muscles are bigger you can hit some poses in the gym as well. Just don't scream when you do so!

Posture

Good posture is a necessity for carrying the skeletal muscles to their best advantage. Bad posture detracts from the appearance of the physique, and good posture enhances it. You don't have to go overboard on posture and look like a Marine drill sergeant, simply keep your chest and chin up, shoulders parallel with the floor, and your stomach tucked in. Good posture is also an advantage in promoting good health.

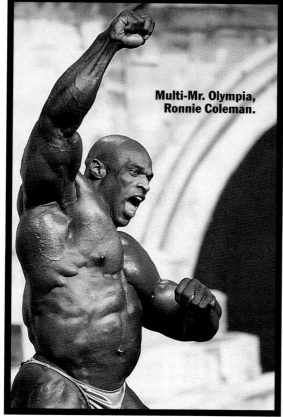

Multi-Mr. Olympia,
Ronnie Coleman.

Contest Preparation

If you do choose to enter a competition, you will need to go through a preparation phase. There are several considerations – diet, training time frame, posing preparation, choice of routine (as well as music), tanning, and even shaving of the body (in order to maximally display the muscles). Diet is perhaps the most important factor in precontest preparation. Dave Spindel points out:"The precontest diet should be approached in such a manner that the athlete is no more than 5 to 10 pounds over his contest weight at least 16 weeks out from the show. The diet should then be geared so that you arrive at your contest weight two weeks prior to your show. If this gradual dieting approach is adopted, you will have time for the skin to thin out (a process that does not happen quickly). Another benefit of this schedule is that you will be able to keep your workout energy at the level it needs to be, since you will not be crash dieting."

The precontest diet approach involves gradually cutting back on calories as the contest draws near. One trick used by some professionals is to cut way down on caloric intake in the final few weeks before the contest, then to have a good intake of carbs right before the show to give the muscles a sudden burst of fullness.

The training intensity is also picked up. This means more ferocious workouts. Spindel notes: In order to expedite the cutting process we can pick up the intensity of training simply by cutting down the rest time between sets. This increased intensity combined with additional posing (30 to 60 minutes per day) will produce the hardness that is the benchmark of the winning contest physique. Training tempo is picked up, with more frequent workouts and often an incorporation of more aerobic work into the mix. The push toward the contest is grueling – more work and less food to fuel the training. Contest preparation is one of the toughest phases of any sport.

The best place to enter your first contest would be in the novice division of a local or regional competition. Titles are contested by locality, by state or region, and there are a variety of national and international competitions in the bodybuilding world. The ultimate climax, the Super Bowl of bodybuilding, are the Mr. and Ms. Olympia competitions, the winner of which receives the title of best bodybuilder in the world. Since its inception in the mid-'60s, only a handful of men have won the prestigious Mr. Olympia, and even fewer women have won the Ms. O since it began in 1980.

Bodybuilding is a sport and art form comprised of several key elements that add up to a larger whole. Consider using them all to fashion a physique that is ultimately the best form of muscularity you can achieve.

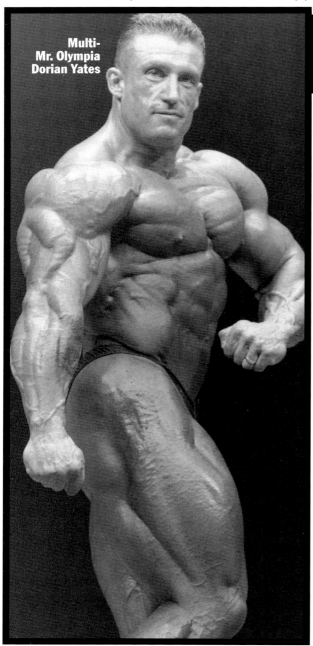

Multi-
Mr. Olympia
Dorian Yates

Thoughts From the Pros on Ancillary Elements

On aerobics: *"Off-season I do aerobics three times a week. I think a small amount of aerobics on a stationary bike or stairstepper, or a fast walk, for example, actually helps recuperation between workouts."*
– Dorian Yates

On posing: *"Bodybuilding is all about displaying lots of high-quality muscle … Pay particular attention to developing a balanced physique before you enter a show."* – Skip La Cour

Pushing it: *"I'm a competitive bodybuilder, and I'm on a journey to see how far I can go in this sport."*
– Chris Cormier

The full package: *"It all comes down to this: If you don't have that mental toughness, that eye of the tiger, then your total fitness package will come unwrapped."*
– Peter Nielsen,
Mr. International Universe

Sources

Smart Exercise by Covert Bailey
ShawnRay.net
Flex, May 2000
Flex, March 1995
Strength and Conditioning Journal, August 2000
Journal of Strength and Conditioning Research, February 2000
www.hugenasserelsonbaty.com
Blood and Guts by Dorian Yates
Essentials of Strength Training and Conditioning
Will of Iron by Peter Nielsen
Muscle & Fitness, June 2000
American Health & Fitness, February 2001
www.hardcorebodybuilding.com
Flex, April 2000
Physical, September 2000
Arnold: The Education of a Bodybuilder
Unleashing the Wild Physique
SpanerFitness online
The 10-Minute Leap
www.drsquat.com – glossary of training and nutrition terms
Lou Ferrigno's Guide to Personal Power, Bodybuilding and Fitness
The Male Bodybuilder Online
MuscleMag, April 1997
jimmymentis.com
Ironman, March 2001
www.skiplacour.com
Avery's Sports Nutrition Almanac
MuscleMag, April 2000
MuscleMag, April 1997
Physical, February 2001
Michael Leveritt and Peter Abernethy, "Effects of Carbohydrate Restriction on Strength Performance," *Journal of Strength and Conditioning Research*
Jean Storlie, "The Art of Refueling," *Training & Conditioning*, April 1998
Haff, Stone, etc., "The Effects of Carbohydrate Supplementation on Multiple Sessions and Bouts of Resistance Exercise," *Journal of Strength and Conditioning Research*, May 1999
Sophie Sjoholm, "Recover Faster … Eat," Sports Afield, November 1999, p.76
Smartbasic.com glossary
Mind & Muscle Power, April 2000
http://www.astaxanthin.org/
http://www.nutritionalsupplements.com/
http://www.lougehrigsdisease.net/als pages/creatine.htm
http://www.healthhelper.com/vitamins/supp/dessicat.htm
http://onhealth.webmd.com/fitness/briefs/reuters/item,87466.asp
JAMA Study on Androstenedione – A Critique by Owen Fonorow
Bill Phillips's *Supplement Review*
Muscle & Fitness, June 2000
Encyclopedia.com
ephedrine-ephedra.com
MuscleMag, 1999 "Back to Basics"
http://www.bodybuilders.com/
http://www.maxsportsmag.com/coverstory/issue13/13cs1.htm
Flex, October 1995
http://www.musclejam.com/_advice/buildmassdiet.html
southfloridamuscle.com
Ironman, February 1996
http://www.leonardfitness.com/prioritytraining.htm
http://members.aol.com/fattalkguy/MuscleMassMyths.html
http://members.tripod.com/Dramo13/Exercises/StripSets.html
http://www.naturalstrength.com/research/high-intens.html
http://www.uers.qwest.net/~buildingmuscle/pre-exhaust.htm
Flex, May 1996
eastcoastmuscle.com
Dispelling the Myths – "A Logical Approach to Contest Preparation" by Dave Spindel (online)
MuscleMag, October 2000

This book is not intended as medical advice, nor is it offered for use in the diagnosis of any health condition or as a substitute for medical treatment and/or counsel. Its purpose is to explore advanced topics on sports nutrition and exercise. All data is for information only. Use of any of the programs within this book is at the sole risk and choice of the reader.

Contributing Photographers

Josef Adlt, Jim Amentler, Alex Ardenti,
Garry Bartlett, John A. Butler, Paula Crane,
Ralph DeHaan, Irvin Gelb, Robert Kennedy,
Chris Lund, Jason Mathas, Mitsuru Okabe,
David Paul, Rick Schaff, Rob Sims, Art Zeller